COVID-19 Responses of Local Communities around the World

Presenting a wide range of international case studies, the contributors to this book study the impact of COVID-19 on the risks faced by communities around the globe.

Examining cases from the Americas, Europe and Asia – including Mexico, Brazil, China, India, France and Belgium – Kuah, Guiheux, Lim and their collaborators look at how communities have coped with the social and economic impacts of the pandemic, as well as the public health concerns. Using a framework of risks, fear and trust, they evaluate how the global health crisis has both revealed and exacerbated a deep crisis of confidence in institutions and systems around the world. In reaction to this they also look at how individuals, social groups and communities have faced fears and built trust at a more local level. The units of spatial analysis in these cases include urban cities, neighborhoods, slum settlements, migrant camps, schools, markets and homes, for a broad spectrum of case types and rich empirical data.

This book is essential reading for social scientists including sociologists, anthropologists and scholars of other disciplines looking to understand the impact of the COVID-19 pandemic internationally and on a multi-scalar level.

Khun Eng Kuah is Distinguished Professor of Anthropology and Chinese Diaspora Studies at the School of International Studies at Jinan University, Guangzhou, China.

Gilles Guiheux is Professor of Sociology of China at the Centre d'Etudes en Sciences Sociales sur les Mondes Africains, Americains et Asiatiques, Université Paris Cité, France.

Francis K. G. Lim is Associate Professor of Sociology at Nanyang Technological University, Singapore.

Routledge Advances in Sociology

345 Recognising Adoptee Relationships
Christine A. Lewis

346 Schools, Space and Culinary Capital
Gurpinder Singh Lalli

347 Academic Freedom and Precarity in the Global North
Free as a Bird
Edited by Aslı Vatansever and Aysuda Kölemen

348 Framing Social Theory
Reassembling the Lexicon of Contemporary Social Sciences
Edited by Paola Rebughini and Enzo Colombo

349 Space, Mobility, and Crisis in Mega-Event Organisation
Tokyo Olympics 2020's Atmospheric Irradiations
Rodanthi Tzanelli

350 Class Boundaries in Europe
The Bourdieusian Approach in Perspective
Edited by Johs. Hjellbrekke, Cédric Hugrée, Étienne Penissat and Alexis Spire

351 COVID-19 Responses of Local Communities around the World
Exploring Trust in the Context of Risk and Fear
Edited by Khun Eng Kuah, Gilles Guiheux and Francis K. G. Lim

352 Remaking Culture and Music Spaces
Affects, Infrastructures, Futures
Edited by Ian Woodward, Jo Haynes, Pauwke Berkers, Aileen Dillane and Karolina Golemo

353 Capitalisms and Democracies
Can Growth and Equality be Reconciled?
Edited by Carlo Trigilia

354 Debates Around Abortion in the Global North
Europe, North America, Canada and Asia
Edited by Fabienne Portier-Le Cocq

For more information about this series, please visit: https://www.routledge.com/Routledge-Advances-in-Sociology/book-series/SE0511

COVID-19 Responses of Local Communities around the World

Exploring Trust in the Context of Risk and Fear

Edited by Khun Eng Kuah, Gilles Guiheux and Francis K. G. Lim

Routledge
Taylor & Francis Group
LONDON AND NEW YORK

First published 2023
by Routledge
4 Park Square, Milton Park, Abingdon, Oxon OX14 4RN

and by Routledge
605 Third Avenue, New York, NY 10158

Routledge is an imprint of the Taylor & Francis Group, an informa business

British Library Cataloguing in Publication Data
A catalogue record for this book is available from the British Library

Library of Congress Cataloging in Publication Data
A catalog record for this book has been requested

ISBN: 978-1-032-27076-0 (hbk)
ISBN: 978-1-032-27077-7 (pbk)
ISBN: 978-1-003-29122-0 (ebk)

DOI: 10.4324/9781003291220

Typeset in Times New Roman
by Deanta Global Publishing Services, Chennai, India

Contents

Figures

Contributors

Álvaro Caballeros is a sociologist at the Universidad de San Carlos de Guatemala and Rafael Landivar University. He graduated from the School of Political Science at the Universidad de San Carlos de Guatemala, and serves as coordinator of the Migration Area of the Instituto de Estudios Interétnicos y de los Pueblos Indígenas. His work deals with migration dynamics, human rights, children and indigenous peoples, rural development and labor migration. He has published several books and scientific papers, has been an active member of civil society organizations for migration, and is a member of the LMI MESO, an international collaboration program between France, Mexico and Central American countries.

Véronique Dupont is a Senior Research Fellow in Urban Studies at the French National Research Institute for Sustainable Development (IRD), in the CESSMA research unit – the Centre for Social Sciences Studies on Africa, America and Asia, Université Paris Cité (France). She is associated with the Centre for Indian and South Asian Studies, Paris and is a senior visiting fellow at the Centre for Policy Research, Delhi. She was joint director of CESSMA from 2014 to 2018, and the director of the Centre for Social Sciences and Humanities of New Delhi from 2003 to 2007. Her research focuses on the socio-spatial transformations of Indian metropolises. She is particularly interested in the interrelations between urban policies and residential and coping strategies of the populations in informal settlements.

Laurent Faret is Professor of Geography at Université Paris Cité. He is a member of the CESSMA (Centre d'études en sciences sociales sur les mondes africains, américains et asiatiques) and former Director of SEDET. His research interests are on international migration dynamics and the related territorial and political transformations, urban dynamics resulting from transit movements and settlement of mobile populations. He is author or editor of books on these themes, among which are *Migrant Protection and the City in the Americas* (2021), *Les circulations transnationales. Lire les turbulences migratoires contemporaines* (2009) and *Migrants des Suds* (2009). He is member of the LMI MESO, an international collaboration Program between France, Mexico and Central American countries.

Chong Gao is Associate Professor in the Department of Sociology at Hong Kong Shue Yan University, Hong Kong. His research interests include sociocultural analysis of old-time brand businesses in China and beyond, corporate community involvement, modernization and Chinese entrepreneurship, business and public health, and others. His publications have appeared in many international journals (e.g., *China Perspectives*, *Human Organization*, *Asian Journal of Social Science*, *International Journal of Entrepreneurship and Small Business*) and in several edited books published by Routledge, Amsterdam University Press and other prestigious publishers. He is writing a book on community involvement activities of time-honored business firms in Guangzhou, China.

M. M. Shankare Gowda is an independent social science researcher based in Delhi. He holds a PhD in political sciences and was a postdoctoral fellow of the Indian Council of Social Sciences Research from 2009 to 2012. He had been associated with the Centre for Policy Research, Delhi. He is now an associated researcher with the Centre for Social Sciences and Humanities (CSH) of New Delhi. His areas of interest include identity politics, government and politics, party system and local and urban governance in India. He has conducted extensive field research in Delhi as well as several states in India.

Gilles Guiheux is Professor at Université Paris Cité (France) and researcher at the Centre for Social Sciences Studies on the African, American and Asian Worlds (CESSMA). He is a senior fellow at the Institut Universitaire de France (IUF). A China specialist, he specializes in economic sociology and sociology of labor. He has recently published *The People's Republic of China* (Polity, 2022) and edited a special issue of *Entreprises et histoire* on the history of socialist enterprises (2021/2). He is currently researching the transformations of China's garment industry. His most recent publication on the subject is "Chinese Worker's Livelihood Strategies: A Zhejiang Case Study in the Garment Industry", *China Perspectives*, 2021/4, 51–59.

Isabelle Hillenkamp is a socioeconomist, researcher at the Research Institute for Development (IRD, France) and member of the Centre for Social Sciences Studies on the African, American and Asian Worlds (CESSMA, Paris). Her research, in Mexico, Bolivia and Brazil has focused on the solidarity economy and agroecology from a gender perspective. She is currently coordinating the ANR project GENgiBRe "Relationship to nature and gender equality: A contribution to critical theory from feminist practices and mobilizations in agroecology in Brazil" (2021–2025). The results of her research have been published in French, English, Portuguese and Spanish academic journals and books.

Hong Jin is an independent researcher based in Shenzhen, China. She earned her PhD from the Department of Sociology, the University of Hong Kong, and worked at Elsevier afterwards. Her research interests include international migration, national and ethnic identities, gender and transnational family. Her current research is on the COVID-19 pandemic, policies and community responses in the Greater Bay Area in China.

Khun Eng Kuah is Distinguished Professor of Anthropology and Chinese Diaspora Studies at the School of International Studies and Academy of Overseas Chinese Studies, Jinan University (Guangzhou, China). Her research specializations include Chinese diaspora–China connections (hometown connections, migration and identity, Chinese entrepreneurship, Chinese women, social and cyber-capital; social movements; China–global Chinese philanthropy; heritage and traditional Chinese medicine and herbal tea) and Reformist Buddhism, Buddhist compassion and philanthropy in East and Southeast Asia. She is the author of five books including one in the Chinese language; editor/co-editor of nine edited books and six special journal issues; and author of around 90 journal articles and book chapters. Her latest book is *The Social Production of Buddhist Compassion in Chinese Society* (Routledge, 2022).

Jingjing Li is a doctoral candidate in social and cultural anthropology at IMMRC, KU Leuven. She is also affiliated with the Department of Applied Linguistics, University of Antwerp, Belgium. Her research focuses on social artistic interventions on urban voids, migration studies and urban social housing.

Francis K.G. Lim is Associate Professor of Sociology at the Nanyang Technological University, Singapore. His research interests revolve around religion in various Asian cultures and societies. He has conducted fieldwork in Nepal, Singapore, Tibet and other parts of China. His latest monograph, *Christianity and Social Engagement in China* (Routledge, 2021) examines how Christians seek to transform China through the workplace, social media and community development work. His other book publications include *Imagining the Good Life: Negotiating Culture and Development in Nepal Himalaya* (Brill, 2008); *Christianity and the State in Asia: Complicity and Conflict* (Routledge, 2009); *Mediating Piety: Technology and Religion in Contemporary Asia* (Brill, 2009); and *Christianity in Contemporary China: Socio-cultural Perspectives* (Routledge, 2013).

Natália Lobo is a Brazilian agroecologist, currently a master's student, affiliated with the Social Sciences Graduate Program on Development, Agriculture and Society at the Federal Rural University of Rio de Janeiro (Brazil). She is currently a collaborator on the ANR project GENgiBRe "Relationship to nature and gender equality. A contribution to critical theory from feminist practices and mobilizations in agroecology in Brazil" (2021–2025). She is particularly interested in topics related to the green economy, financialization of nature and feminism.

Olga Odgers-Ortiz is Professor at El Colegio de la Frontera Norte, located at the Mexico–US border. She received her PhD in Sociology (1998) from the École des Hautes Études en Sciences Sociales (Paris, France). Her work is centered on the relationship between religion and international migration in the Central America/Mexico/US migratory field. Within this field, she is interested in religious practices and health. She is a member of the LMI MESO, an international collaboration program between France, Mexico and Central American countries.

Ching Lin Pang is Associate Professor in the Department of Applied Linguistics, Translation and Interpreting and Academic Director of the Postgraduate Program China Europe Cultural Curatorship Studies, University of Antwerp, Belgium. She is also affiliated with KU Leuven, Belgium. Her research is situated at the intersection of mobilities, multilingualism, arts and aesthetics of cultural workers in the urban context. She is the editor of the "China Matters" series, Leuven University Press. She is an editorial member of Leuven University Press and the *Cosmopolitan Civil Societies Journal*.

María Teresa Rodríguez López has been a Researcher and Professor at CIESAS-Golfo (Centro de Investigaciones y Estudios Superiores en Antropología Social) since 1994 and a member of the Mexican National System of Researchers since 1998. She holds a PhD in anthropology from the Universidad Autónoma Metropolitana, Unidad Iztapalapa, Mexico. Her areas of interest include issues related to ethnic identities, religion, family dynamics and indigenous and Central American migrations. She is the author of books, articles and chapters on these topics. She is a member of the LMI MESO, an international collaboration program between France, Mexico and Central American countries.

Beatriz Schwenck is a Brazilian sociologist, currently a PhD student, affiliated with the Postgraduate Program in Sociology at the University of Campinas (Brazil) and the Centre for Social Sciences Studies on the African, American and Asian Worlds of the Université Paris Cité (France). She is the beneficiary of an ARTS PhD scholarship from the Research Institute for Development (IRD, France). She is particularly interested in topics related to the solidarity economy and feminism.

Ziying You is Associate Professor of Chinese Studies at the College of Wooster (Ohio, US). Her research interests include Chinese literature, folklore studies, food studies, mythology and popular religion, critical heritage studies, women's, gender and sexuality studies, anti-Asian racism and public health. She is the author of *Folk Literati, Contested Tradition, and Heritage in Contemporary China: Incense Is Kept Burning* (Indiana University Press, 2020). She is co-editor of *Chinese Folklore Studies Today: Discourse and Practice* (2019) and of a special issue for the journal *Asian Ethnology*, titled *Intangible Cultural Heritage in Asia: Traditions in Transition* (2020).

Qiaoyun Zhang is an Assistant Professor of the Department of Social Sciences at Beijing Normal University-Hong Kong Baptist University United International College, China. A cultural anthropologist, Dr. Zhang's research interests include post-disaster recovery, risk and culture, ethnic relations and intangible cultural heritage safeguarding in China. She has produced more than ten publications in leading peer-reviewed journals and edited volumes. Her research has been funded by major research grants in China and the United States. Currently, Dr. Zhang is researching how different societies adapt to the COVID-19 pandemic based on specific sociocultural mapping of risk.

Preface

The declaration of the new coronavirus SARS-CoV2, also known as COVID-19, as a pandemic and a public health hazard has led to intensive actions on all fronts, from the scientific understanding of the origin of the virus to the medical and pharmaceutical chase for a vaccine to social sciences research in understanding the roles of the governments and society in the management and governance of the COVID-19 virus. Amidst these research activities, our edited book is concerned with the local community and how different local communities in the global world negotiate the fear of the COVID-19 virus together with the trust and mistrust of the state and society in dealing and managing this virus as well as the types of network structures that the local communities created to foster relationships to cope with this ongoing pandemic.

This edited book began with an online international workshop on the "Responses of local communities to COVID-19: exploring issues of trust in the context of risk and fear" held in December 2020. The editors are grateful to their respective institutions, namely Jinan University (Guangzhou, China), Université Paris Cité (France) and Nanyang Technological University (Singapore) for the support that they have provided. The workshop would not have been successful without the participation of scholars from different parts of the world who were researching the various COVID-19 issues confronting the local communities in Asia, Europe and the North and Latin and Central Americas. After the successful workshop, the editors worked collaboratively with the participating scholars to ensure that all chapters addressed the central theoretical concerns of this book and attained a high academic standard for publication purposes. The editors are also grateful to Simon Bates at Routledge and his editorial team for assisting them in bringing this edited book to fruition.

Finally, the editors would like to thank their respective families and loved ones for the support they provided that enabled us to complete this project in good time and with joy.

Conducting research on the pandemic was a way of distancing ourselves from it during what were sometimes difficult times, particularly during periods of lockdowns while we were confined to our domestic spaces. At the same time, conducting rigorous and innovative research also allowed us to not give in to our emotions. We would like to dedicate this edited book to all those who have helped in one way or another to make life a bit easier for all of us who have to live under the shadows of the COVID-19 pandemic.

Khun Eng Kuah, Gilles Guiheux and Francis K. G. Lim
April 2022

1 Negotiating trust, risk and fear during the COVID-19 pandemic

Responses within local communities across the world

Khun Eng Kuah[1]*, Gilles Guiheux and Francis K.G. Lim*

Introduction

The world has been afflicted with the COVID-19 infection since late 2019 and by January 2020 it was declared a health emergency of public concern and a pandemic. By spring 2022, the world has witnessed six waves of different strains of COVID-19 infections. Since the World Health Organization (WHO) declared it a pandemic, countries throughout the world have adopted a range of strategies to bring this infection under control. Two years since the infection was first detected, the world is coming to terms with it, with many countries adopting policies of coexisting with the virus despite the continued outbreaks of this infectious illness.

Who to trust and rely on in times of the pandemic? This is the central question addressed by this book. The COVID-19 crisis, as a public health pandemic, effectively restructured the sentence that revealed the interplay of trust and mistrust among the various players involved in the crisis and its mitigation: individuals, families, various types of social groups, but also corporations or civil organizations, as well as state institutions on different levels – from the local to the national. This introductory chapter provides a general perspective on how the issue of trust is articulated in the local community in response to the COVID-19 pandemic. It starts with a review of the chronology, from the emergence of the pandemic to its global spread, and the varying measures taken by states to address the crisis. In the second part, this chapter reflects on the scale of analysis: that of local communities. In the third part, it explores the concepts of risk and trust. The introduction ends with an outline of the different chapters of the book.

The COVID-19 pandemic

In late 2019, when SARS-CoV-2 – subsequently known as COVID-19 – was identified as the infectious virus that had spread throughout the world, the origin was suspected as being a wholesale seafood market in Wuhan. This was the Wuhan Huanan Sea Food Wholesale Market (武汉华南海鲜批发市场). In addition to selling seafood, this wholesale market also sold an array of wild and live animals including snakes, rodents and raccoon dogs. Earlier scientific studies

DOI: 10.4324/9781003291220-1

have pointed to bats as a plausible incubator and transmitter of COVID-19 from animal to human. However, recent studies by various scientific groups have pinpointed a raccoon dog as a possible index transmitter (*Nature News*, 27/2/2022).[2]

From Wuhan city to the global world

The rapid spread and the severity of the highly transmissible COVID-19 infection soon led to a complete lockdown of Wuhan city where residents were confined to their households and movements in and out of the city were restricted to only those that provided essential goods and services. This rapid and complete lockdown of a city with a population of 11 million people was unprecedented in China and created shockwaves across continents. China's policy was to eliminate this infectious virus at all costs. As the virus spread across the world, other countries started to follow suit with lockdowns and closed borders.

From the initial discovery of COVID-19 in Wuhan, the virus rapidly spread across the world, first to America and Europe, then to Asia and later to Africa. As of March 2022, there were 452 million cases of infection globally; the United States was the country with the most infections, totaling over 79 million infected. Closely following behind the US were India and Brazil, with 43 million infected and close to 30 million infected, respectively. Deaths from COVID-19 infections stood at over six million globally.[3] The daily infection rate continued to rise until the beginning of 2022 when the population of countries that had been given three doses of vaccines started experiencing a plateau and a gradual decline in infection rate.[4]

From lockdowns and mask wearing to vaccination

The WHO has recommended strategies to prevent cross-infection of COVID-19 through the wearing of masks, social distancing, restricting the size of social gatherings and tracking the movements of people. With the recommendation of mask wearing and a world population of 7.9 billion, there is a severe shortage of masks worldwide. But, crucially, it has also reflected global inequalities where the wealthier developed nations were able to produce and purchase masks at the expense of the developing countries. At the same time, it has also led to the politics of mask production, procurement and gifting. China, as the greatest mask production country, was able to cash in on the global demands and at the same time engaged in what some scholars regarded as "mask diplomacy". The term "mask diplomacy" refers to China's shipments of masks, personal protective equipment and medical resources to developing countries as well as some developed nations such as Canada, South Korea and others. Because Canada is a developed country, "mask diplomacy" became part of the foreign policy used to negotiate with the Canadian government over the sanctions imposed on Huawei and the arrest of the CFO of Huawei (*All FSI News/Blog*, 16/6/2020).[5] Other developed nations also provided masks and other medical supplies to the developing world, but their efforts were criticized by the WHO as minuscule and not reaching the neediest parts of the world.

Since the COVID-19 outbreak, big biopharmaceutical firms and research institutes have been working on a vaccine. Today, there are two types of vaccine. One uses the genetic approach that uses DNA and mRNA to produce the non-inactivated vaccine (nucleic acid vaccines), while the second uses the traditional whole microbe approach that produces inactivated vaccines.[6] Western biopharmaceutical firms and research labs worked to produce the nuclei acid vaccine while Mainland Chinese firms produced the inactivated vaccine. Large western biopharmaceutical firms like Pfizer-BioNTech (Comirnaty), AstraZeneca (Oxford), Moderna and Johnson & Johnson have started producing mRNA vaccines and obtained emergency use authorization. The WHO worked with various partners to produce the vaccines for global use and monitored the effectiveness and side effects of the new vaccines.[7]

The WHO has recommended vaccinations to stop the spread of COVID-19. Almost all countries have adopted this recommendation and started vaccinating their population in 2020. By March 2022, wealthy nations have reached over 90% fully vaccinated rates of citizens while poorer developing nations have vaccination rates of well below 50% of their population.[8] African countries have little access to the vaccine because of the cost incurred in procurement. This has led to the WHO's criticism of global vaccine inequality and the call for more equitable distribution of vaccines to the developing world. The WHO's argument is that the world needs to be protected to ensure that all are safe from COVID-19 infections and to stop rapid mutations of the virus into other strains.

Free COVID-19 vaccinations have been given to the citizens by the governments of the nation states and most countries did not adopt a mandatory approach to the vaccination but strongly encouraged it. In western liberal countries, while a large segment of the population followed vaccination directives and was vaccinated, a small portion protested the use of vaccination. These were the anti-vaxxers or vaccine deniers who organized protests against COVID-19 vaccinations, while those in developing nations had little access to the vaccines.

From providing the first dose of vaccination to the third booster jab, United Kingdom has been instrumental in pushing a high vaccination rate to achieve "herd immunity" among its population. The WHO defined "herd immunity" as the indirect protection from an infectious disease either through natural transmission of the infection from person to person or through vaccination until a majority of the population has acquired immunity that will stop further spread of the infectious disease. It further recommended that "herd immunity" be attained through vaccination in order to lower the chance of severe illness and unnecessary deaths arising from COVID-19 infections.[9] As a result of this recommendation, most countries have vigorously pushed for vaccination of their populations. However, the COVID-19 virus has mutated. The emergence of the Delta strain of the virus greatly impacted medical and hospital resources, as its severity resulted in an even greater number of deaths globally. This hastened the vaccination rate and the decision to encourage a second vaccine dose. Yet again, in 2021, with the discovery of the Omicron strain and its rapid transmission rate, countries throughout the world insisted on giving their citizens a third dose of the vaccine. Several countries have now made two booster doses available to citizens too. However, this further reflected the inequality of vaccine distribution as at this time in Africa, less than 10% of the population were fully vaccinated.[10]

With the high vaccination rate across developed regions, the world is now gradually "opening up" and countries in the western world and parts of Asia are reopening their borders. Across Europe and America, the nation states have removed the barriers of social distancing, size of group gatherings and masking. Further, they have also implemented vaccinated travel lanes and subsequently removed this and implemented open border as well as removed compulsory hotel and home quarantines for travelers. Asian countries also began to follow suit in an attempt to reignite their travel industries and economies that were badly affected by border closures.

The spread of COVID-19 infections within individual countries across the world has greatly impacted the social and economic life of the individuals within the boundary of the nation-state. This has created a humanitarian crisis of global proportion that affected individuals, families and businesses. Wealthier countries have poured funds into their economies to help businesses and individuals who were affected by the lockdowns and retrenchments. Despite this, individuals and families at the lower end of the economic scale were still badly affected at the local community level. This is even more crucial for developing countries where there is less state-level assistance provided. As such, those who have fallen through the cracks have increasingly become dependent on international and local charitable organizations and NGOs for assistance, even with their daily needs including food supplies. Food insecurity has become an acute problem. According to a think tank for food, Foodtank, the Global FoodBanking Network reported that during this period of the COVID-19 pandemic, requests for food have gone up by 132% from 2019 to 2020. It is estimated that in 2020, there was an increase of 320 million people facing moderate to severe food insecurity. Food banks have become an important humanitarian pillar to help with relief efforts for individuals and families in the local communities, particularly those outside the reach of the state.[11]

When COVID-19 infections started spreading rapidly, there were fears within local communities as they wrestled with their responses to this pandemic. This was an unknown virus. There was confusion at all levels in implementing policies and strategies to cope with the transmission of infections. Individuals and local communities had to contend with the issues of fear, risks and trust in the policies, strategies and actions of their government. From lockdowns to social distancing and mask wearing, there were confusion and resistance among a segment of the population. The introduction of COVID-19 vaccination has compounded the fear and risks experienced by the individuals in their local community. There was a high level of distrust of the effectiveness of social distancing and mask wearing as people continued to be infected with the COVID-19 virus. The COVID-19 vaccine – which is a new vaccine that was approved for use under the emergency use authorization – has created an even higher level of fear and distrust given that the side effects of the vaccine are still an unknown factor.

In light of all this, individuals also responded pro-actively, and in unique ways, in their local communities. Some worked in tandem with their government's policies and strategies, while others acted in line with local and global NGOs to assist their community in times of need. Yet, there are others who worked independently and in small groups to help their communities cope. How the individuals and local communities work and respond to the COVID-19 pandemic is highly dependent on how they view risks and experience fear in this global pandemic and the extent to which they trust their government in response to this global pandemic.

The concept of community

For methodological reasons, surveys were carried out with various communities. In this section, we explore communities as spatial units of analysis comprised of local neighborhood districts, townships, vernacular/language schools, local migrant community groups, refugee groups and slums. The concept of community was born, along with sociology, from the great upheavals that marked the 18th and 19th centuries: political revolutions in America and France, the industrial revolution in Great Britain and later in the rest of Europe. In his book *Community and Society*, first published in 1887, F. Tönnies, the founder of community theory, constructs the famous dichotomy of *gemeinschaft* versus Gesellschaft. The community is characterized by the affective and spatial proximity of individuals. It is thus defined as a "community of blood, place and spirit" where the whole takes precedence over the individual. On the other hand, society is the scene of forced individualism, of generalized competition between individuals who are now separated; self-interest is now the basis of all social relations, which tend to be reduced to contractualized exchanges. The concepts of community and society thus represent the two antithetical poles of an evolving social reality. According to Tönnies, the disintegration of *gemeinschaft* allows the advent of capitalism. Although history favors the development of Gesellschaft, the two systems can coexist.

An extensive social sciences literature has analyzed the decline of solidarities and increasing individualism in modern societies, but the notion that there was a golden age of traditional community life has been destroyed by historians and cultural theorists (Stone 1977; Williams 1973). Recently, one side of the debate took the form of anxiety about the decline of social capital and the fragmentation of face-to-face community rooted in place (Putnam 2000) and the other side, a celebration of the increasing "disembeddeness" of individuals and families, and the potential that this creates for individualization, choice, negotiation and democratic relationships (Giddens 1992; Beck 1992). This has implication for trust. Typically, social trust is prevalent in face-to-face communities, while system trust is prevalent in highly differentiated societies. Empirically, both are present, to varying degrees.

Community studies

Community studies designate prolific literature carried out on villages and social isolates. Among the most famous are W. Loyd Warner's *Yankee City Series*

(1941–1949), looking at a small American town, Newburyport, and William F. Whyte's *Street Corner Society*, describing an Italian slum in Boston (1943). In *Communities in Britain: Social Life in Town and Country* (1966), R. Frankenberg brings together the findings of some of the most influential field studies undertaken in Britain in the mid-1960s. The village, the market town, the urban housing estate and sections of great cities are examined successively, revealing the power structures, the degree of communality or isolation, and the relationship patterns prevailing in different environments. Here is Frankenberg's definition of a community: "those who live in a community have overriding economic interests which are the same or complementary … Their common interest in things give them a common interest in each other" (Frankerberg 1966: 238).

Community studies declined in the 1970s and 1980s in the context of the growing centrality of social class in sociological analysis. The focus of interest shifted to the regional, national and international levels. Local communities were no longer held in command of their own economic and political fate, if they ever were. Thus, what could be explained by studying local social relations *per se* was severely limited. Larger institutional structures were the overriding concern. The shift in attention to regional political economy and beyond, of course, obliterated the study of local social structure. In a famous article, Manuel Castells, for instance, argued that a city is not a social entity (Castells 1968).

Yet community studies and locality studies are not dead. If the rural–urban continuum is in disgrace, there is still much interest in contemporary social sciences to the local versus the national. The emphasis is less on the study of "community" as such and more on the study of the primary groups – whether made up of neighbors, friends or kin, for instance (Bulmer 1985). Recently, sociology has been actively researching the primary group of ties. The perspective is not studying settlement patterns but social networks and how people construct their relationships (Bidard and Lavenu 2005). The approach is formulated in terms of social networks rather than geographical space.

There was also rehabilitation of the community as a theoretical concept in the 1980s. Its revival concentrated on the way communities, national and local, were imagined (Anderson 1983), and on local communities as symbolic constructions (Cohen 1985). This perspective emphasized how people define and attach meanings to their community that serve to include and exclude the insiders and outsiders. The research explored how particular communities were constituted. The idea that people use symbols as a resource to reassert the boundaries of communities is particularly useful to understand how trust evolves in a time of crisis.

Community as a methodological strategy

In this volume, community study is understood as a method of empirical investigation. Communities are understood as "on-going systems of interaction, usually within a locality, that have some degree of permanence" (Bell and Newby 1971); they are open systems. To understand social change during the COVID-19 pandemic, we look at how people have been affected in a particular place at a particular time. We share R. Frankenberg's claim that the best way to understand general social processes is through the study of their manifestation in the details of social life (Frankenberg 1990; Nicke and Aull Davies 2005). Communities can be seen as a site to test general theories on trust and mistrust.

Diverse communities are considered in this book. Gao and Kuah's chapter examines kin and friend networks in the Hong Kong context. The term is also used in a geographical sense. "Community" is defined in terms of a village, part of a street, a housing estate or an established residential area covering several streets. Communities are here defined by place, in contrast to other places. Dupont and Gowda look at two Delhi sites where former residents of a large slum have been relocated. Guiheux analyzes a locale in the Paris suburbs where a large wholesale market is based; the community gathers a group of people in a specific activity located on a limited territory. Kuah and Jin explore the residents of two local residents' communities in Shenzhen and one in Guangzhou, in the south of China, and how they respond to state-directed strategies and actions.

In the book, "community" also designates those who use it in some emotional sense and who stress a "sense of belonging". In that case, "community" is also defined in relation to others and often involves dimensions of identity such as class, faith or ethnicity. In the two Delhi sites looked at by Dupont and Gowda, there were actually several communities based on caste, religion or region of origin and, during the pandemic, solidarity followed pre-existing community-based channels. Guiheux's community is as much a geographical as a social space, as most businessmen share a common Chinese ethnicity. Li and Pang studied Chinese communities in Belgium; how, in the time of the COVID crisis, their trust in the host and home society adjusted. The authors' fieldwork was done at a school which is, at the same time, a geographical and social space. Zhang and You investigated the behavior of another Chinese community in the American state of Florida, by adopting a similar methodology, basing their inquiry on the observation of a volunteer group organized under the leadership of a local Chinese language school. In these two last cases, the community may also be considered as an imagined community built on ethnicity.

Another way in which contributors talk about belonging to a community is in terms of formal membership of organizations. Hillenkamp, Schwenck and Lobo examine how two Brazilian women's organizations have reacted to the pandemic. They look at how solidarity networks have adjusted in relation to local communities and the state. In the case of the chapter by Faret, Odgers, Rodriguez and Caballeros, the community is transnational; the four authors consider a number of social groups and actors – family networks as well as NGOs – that support international migrants between Mexico and the United States.

Diverse territorial and social communities are analyzed by various authors; the networks social actors build on to get through the pandemic crisis and whom they trust and distrust are examined. One shared conclusion in several chapters is that communities are not static or neatly bounded entities that remain constant before, during and after a disaster or crisis (Barrios 2014). Rather, communities are constantly evolving, shaped by powerful social, political and economic forces. Another conclusion is that claims that families and individuals are disembedded and that "traditional" communities are disappearing would seem, at the very least, not to be universally applicable. Communities, notably those rooted in close-knit networks of kin and friends, are still very much in evidence, and this has implications for trust relations.

The concepts of risks and trusts

The COVID-19 pandemic has forced us to ask some difficult questions concerning the foundations of our social and political life. Since it is invisible to the naked eye and its material presence is not easily determined, the SARS-CoV-2 virus generates intense uncertainty and deep ambiguity in many aspects of social interactions that we have previously taken for granted. One of the most fundamental questions that arise is who can be trusted to enter and inhabit our intimate or significant spaces such as the home, community and the nation.

Beck's work on the emergence of "risk society" as a contemporary phase of social history makes the distinction between "natural hazard" and "manufactured risk". Ideal typically, the former was predominant in the so-called pre-modern era where hazards were experienced as naturally occurring. In the modern era, rapid technological advances have reached such high levels of complexity that they often are beyond the complete understanding and effective management of the individuals and institutions that utilize them. This has resulted in what Beck calls the "latent side effects" of technology which, over time, become more problematic, lethal and global:

> the distribution of social problems or "bads" becomes global rather than being limited to local areas or sections of society; in this way the rich and powerful are as much afflicted by the "democratic" impact of risks as more marginalized groups, with the former experiencing the "boomerang effects" of technological developments coming back to haunt them, in contrast to previous eras where money could buy insulation from danger.
>
> (Beck 1992: 7)

While scientists are still debating the actual origins of SARS-CoV-2 virus, we may consider the pandemic as both a natural hazard and manufactured risk. So far, the consensus among many scientists is that the original virus jumped from a host animal to humans via the food chain. As such, the virus may be regarded as a kind of natural hazard. However, the resulting global spread of the virus can be considered an example of a manufactured risk as different complex, abstract expert systems seek to understand it, contain its transmission and mitigate its devastating health impacts on people around the world, in various stages of failure and success. What the pandemic has starkly demonstrated is that Beck's notion of risk society is not just applicable to the so-called developed, highly industrialized societies but also to societies at different stages of development, from Angola to Brazil, from China to Fiji. If risk society is a feature of this present phase of modernity, then what the global nature of the pandemic crisis reveals is that we are all "moderns" now, to paraphrase Bruno Latour.

The studies of different local communities from diverse geographical regions contained in this volume remind us that, when faced with risk, the feelings of anxiety, vulnerability and uncertainty in society are experienced universally. In their own ways, but often in constant interactions with one another through translocal and transnational networks, as local communities find ways to reduce uncertainty and vulnerability, the issue of trust and mistrust becomes all the more salient (Beck 1992; Giddens 1991; Brown and Calnan 2012).

How can we conceptualize trust (and mistrust) when even our most significant social relations (such as parents, children and loved ones) are now feared because they may be infected and infectious, and hence to be spatially segregated through quarantine and "safe distancing" measures? At the same time, we also observe that certain marginalized groups (such as migrant workers and minorities) in society are experiencing heightened discrimination, physical violence and other forms of mistreatment because they are not trusted by the majority or powerful groups who positioned themselves as custodians of the wellbeing of the nation.

Varieties of trust

Definitions of trust in scholarly literature can be broadly categorized into either functional or substantive definitions (for in-depth discussion, see, e.g., Misztal 1996; Hardin 2002; Hosking 2014; Frederiksen 2014). A good example of a functional definition is provided by Luhmann. He conceptualizes trust as an act essential "for the reduction of a future characterized by more or less indeterminate complexity" and involves "the taking of a risk" (Luhmann 2017: 17, 79). For Luhmann, trust is not just a psychological coping mechanism but also a social action, with intersubjectivity as its basis (Frederiksen 2014; Kroeger 2019). Like trust, distrust also functions to reduce complexity. According to Luhmann, both trust and distrust involve generalizations. The former allows social actors to form positive expectations while the latter to form negative expectations. To Luhmann,

> Anyone who does not trust must, therefore, turn to functionally equivalent strategies for the reduction of complexity in order to be able to define a practically meaningful situation at all. He must hone his expectations into negative ones, and so must, in certain respects, become distrustful.
>
> (Luhmann 2017: 79)

In contrast, Newton adopts a substantive definition of trust: it is "the belief that others will not deliberately or knowingly do us harm, if they can avoid it, and will look after our interests, if this is possible" (Newton 2007: 343). In combining both functional and substantive approaches for a more comprehensive definition, we can define trust as a risk-taking act that reduces life's future complexity, based on the belief that others will not deliberately or knowingly do us harm and will look after our interests.

As a broad concept, trust can be further distinguished into different types. First, there is particularized trust or social trust, usually found in communities or groups with strong social bonds underpinned by common values, interests or worldviews. This kind of trust comprises like-minded people who interact closely with and are dependent upon one another (Williams 1988; Newton 2007). Typically, these closely bonded groups tend to have a relatively homogenous culture with powerful social sanctions. Members are socialized into a common culture and strive to forge strong in-group identities. For members of such groups, legitimate authority lies in individuals or entities that are seen as best embodying the values, norms and worldview of the group. While group members tend to trust one another, they are less trustful of people in the out-groups (Gambetta 1988; cf. Douglas and Wildavsky 1982, on sectarian groups).

The other kind of trust that concerns us here is system trust, where social systems (e.g., political, medical, technological, economic) are the objects of trust. This entails that the trustor "assumes that a system is functioning and places his trust in that function and not in … people" (Luhmann 2017:55). Typically, characteristics of system trust include independence from individual motivation (e.g., trust in money) and the requirement of expert knowledge to exercise control over it. System trust exists in complex relationships with particularized, interpersonal trust, and can both substitute and complement each other (Kroeger 2019:166). As Luhmann (2017:58) asks, "Does one trust the chemist, or his assistant, or the doctor, or is it medicine, science or technology?"

All social actors are simultaneously embedded within both personal networks and systems. To varying degrees, both shape people's meaning-making efforts and their social actions. Examples of personal networks are those of the immediate family and wider kin groups, intimate acquaintances, friends, religious or spiritual communities, voluntary associations, interest groups and political parties. At the same time, individuals and their social networks are embedded within systems that are ideal typically underpinned by impersonal rules and norms, highly abstract and technical knowledge, or formal rationality. Such systems include the political and economic systems, highly specialized professions, and state bureaucracies.

Theoretical pluralism: multiple dimensionalities of trust, risk and fear

On the theoretical approaches of this volume, we undertake what may be called "theoretical pluralism" in this collection of a wide variety of empirical cases. Given the multiple dimensionalities of trust, risk and fear in diverse local communities as they confront the pandemic, we refrain from using a single grand theory or framework to arbitrarily impose a kind of false unity or systematic coherence to all the cases presented by the authors. Of course, each contributor may use particular theoretical frameworks that they find useful in analyzing their empirical data. We seek to let the individual cases "speak for themselves", as they were. This is in line with what we consider a key contribution of this collection: socio-anthropological insights into how different local communities at the sub-state levels in various parts of the world respond to the disruptions caused by the pandemic, and how they understand and deal with issues of risk and blame. In short, we think that diverse responses call for diverse theoretical approaches. Heuristically, each contributor may choose to use the theoretical approaches that can best provide analytical insights into specific contexts and situations.

For example, Dupont and Gowda's chapter in this volume examines COVID responses of displaced slum dwellers in Delhi, India, broadly utilizing the distinction between a system-based trust and interpersonal trust as proposed by Giddens and Luhmann. As the coronavirus swept through India and unleashed its devastations on both personal health and social order, the residents of the Kathputli Colony were temporarily resettled in a transit camp. In addressing the question, "whom to trust and to rely on" in these challenging times, the authors have found it useful to further explore Spire's conceptions of symbolic confidence and practical trust as sub-sets of system-based trust. As the authors note, the interaction between symbolic confidence and practical trust allows them to "better understand the distrust entrenched in most of our respondents of certain state institutions as well as some of their seemingly contradictory appreciations of the government measures during India's prolonged lockdown".

This volume's global focus on the responses of local communities includes various migrant communities around the world. In their chapter on the experience of migrants from mainland China in Belgium, Li and Pang want to underscore the importance of examining the dynamic nature of trust relationships in the context of migration and the pandemic. Specifically, they wish to explore how the Chinese immigrants in Belgium negotiate their trust relationships with both their home and host country. To what extent do China's much more draconian and restrictive approaches to curb the spread of the virus affect Chinese immigrants' attitude toward Belgian's relatively less restrictive COVID policies? Does the awareness and experience among Chinese immigrants of policies in their home country influence their levels of trust in their host country?

To answer these questions, Li and Pang provide a critical review of two perspectives on the origin of trust. On the one hand, the cultural theory of trust postulates that trust is learned through an individual's socialization experience from youth in a specific cultural context. This means that one's general disposition toward trust and distrust tends to be relatively stable even in changing circumstances in later life stages. On the other hand, the experiential theory of trust origin emphasizes how changing social and cultural contexts exert a more significant impact on an individual's attitude toward trust relationships.

In other words, one's attitude toward trust relationships can evolve depending on the specific contexts. Researchers utilizing the cultural theory tend to find immigrants' trust in their home country to be relatively stable, and their trust does not seem to be extended to the same extent to their host country. Conversely, some studies in international migration have suggested that migrants' trust adapts to the host country's levels of trust. From their study of the Chinese immigrant community in Belgium, Li and Pang argue that the dichotomy between the two perspectives has often presented too simplified an understanding of the actual experiences of international migrants. Instead, following Isaeva et al. (2015), they adopt an interpretive, context-specific perspective on trust to argue that "trust is not universal and definitive … nor is it a choice between home or host country but rather context-based and encompassing evolving practices and processes".

The pandemic has profoundly impacted various types and transactions of businesses worldwide. Given that trust is central to the conduct of business, it is essential to explore how local business communities and their clients have cultivated and maintained trust with one another. Guiheux's contribution to this volume delves into the complexity of business trust in a wholesale market on the outskirt of Paris, France. In Guiheux's analysis, business trust is inextricably linked with confidence. According to Simmel (1964) and Sellerberg (1982), confidence in modern societies is predicated on non-personal information and institutions such as laws and contracts. Therefore, in developed industrial societies, the execution of business transactions is based more on institutional conditions and less on personal trust.

It is important to note that trust should be considered a process that can develop from low to high trust, starting with small transactions with relatively little risk involved. This allows business partners to demonstrate their trustworthiness over time and then further expand their business ties. Guiheux's chapter also investigates how confidence and trust can be established in online business transactions between complete strangers who are unable to meet in person due to mobility restrictions in the pandemic. This case study of the wholesalers has further illustrated that the rapidly increasing digitization of the economy has facilitated the inexorable rise of a new digital platform-mediated trust (Mohlmann and Geissinger 2018). This takes the form of "peer ratings, reviews, and connections between peers' profile with other social media networks".

The uncertainties posed by the threats of COVID-19

In this volume, our general understanding of how societies dealt with the coronavirus outbreak relates not only to simply hygiene or biomedical science. Crucially, how a society or community views the virus as a threat, determines the risk it poses and enacts the measures to contain the threats and mitigate the risk are seen as inextricably related to how its symbolic system constructs social boundaries, imposes meanings, attributes blame and legitimizes sociopolitical actions. In other words, we want to examine and interrogate a society's symbolic system to understand how it comprehends and deals with both the social and biomedical aspects of the pandemic.

As we underscore how local communities symbolically construct the threats associated with COVID-19, and how the virus is seen as an anomaly, we need to examine how the local community culture constructs the notion of risk and threat.

This is because a community or society's culture comprises a system of symbols and values that allow its members to attribute meanings to events and occurrences they face (Geertz 2000). In this sense, culture mediates the experience of individuals while providing fundamental categories and patterns that impose an order on ideas and values. Given that the culture of a local community acts as a classificatory system and as an important source of meaning, any novel or unprecedented event (e.g., COVID-19) becomes an anomaly that the local community must confront, seek to understand and find ways to manage (Douglas 2002).

Often, that which is anomalous poses a threat and danger to an existing order. Thus, in this instance, the novel coronavirus was deemed "dangerous" from the perspective of existing order of medical knowledge which did not have the adequate expertise to understand and control it. The virus could also be perceived and experienced as a risk and danger to a social order whose relations and structures were struggling to devise new ways to confront it.

From a cultural perspective, a local community may deal with the anomalous event of the initial spread of SARS-CoV-2 in a few ways. First, the local community may seek to reduce ambiguity by subscribing to one or more authoritative interpretations. Here, as Luhmann, Beck and Gidden's works have demonstrated, trust becomes highly salient. Individuals may find interpretations promulgated by fellow members within their social networks to be particularly convincing. For example, a religious group may interpret the meaning of the pandemic in terms of divine actions. Group members may then engage in some efforts to manage the existence of the anomalous virus. As scientific knowledge may not be the primary source of meaning for them, members may continue their religious activities while downplaying or ignoring the various safety measures suggested by the public health authorities. In another scenario, the group members may also consider the virus a serious health risk and avoid certain behaviors, but their interpretation of the threat and risk may differ from that of the medical profession. In this example, with the pandemic understood symbolically in religious terms, the group may conduct rites such as ritual cleansing, divination, healing, etc. to mitigate or counter the perceived risks. However, as Francis Lim argues in his contribution to this volume, in any individual or social group at any particular moment, multiple cultural frameworks may exist with relative degrees of legitimacy that act as sources of trust and mistrust, shaping potential responses and social actions.

Outline of the book

The richness of this edited volume is reflected in each chapter that deals with critical issues of risk, trust and fear from different perspectives. Chapter 2 introduces a broad comparative perspective of the interconnection of trust, risk and blame. Building on the existing social sciences literature on trust, Lim proposes the concept of trust liminality to analyze how the pandemic has resulted in a momentary suspension of trust in different contexts. He presents a theoretical model comprising interactions of particularized and system trust that produce four modalities of social action. The model gives insights into the interactions between trust, risk and fear in individuals and social groups and provides a common analytical framework that can be used to compare different cases across societies and scales.

The two chapters by Gao and Kuah and Kuah and Jin, through ethnographic studies, explore the inter-relationship of the local and state actors and the community responses to the COVID-19 policies. Gao and Kuah examine food consumption patterns in Hong Kong; they argue that trust in people and trust in business played a critical role in enabling consumers to practice safe eating. The strategic use of "thick" interpersonal trust and "thin" trust in business helped reduce ambiguity allowing safe food consumption. Kuah and Jin's chapter focus on two local residential communities in Guangdong province, south of China. They explore how the residents negotiated and constructed compliance with the state-directed strategies and actions. From the initial trust deficit, the public shifted to trust toward the Chinese authorities in the management of the pandemic.

Another perspective advances the idea of how local communities build upon their social networks and trust in their communities to counteract the fear brought upon by COVID-19. These are the chapters by Dupont and Gowda, Hillenkamp et al. and Guiheux. Dupont and Gowda are looking at a population of relocated slum dwellers in Delhi (India). They examine the multidimensional impact of the sanitary and economic crisis and the communities' responses. They argue that solidarity preferentially followed community-based channels. Hillenkamp, Schwenck and Lobo offer a case study of the reactions of two solidarity networks of subaltern women in Brazil. They examine the reorganization of these networks for the ensured continuity of economic practice and mutual aid, the nature of the relations mobilized and their connection to other levels of protection from local communities and the state. Guiheux provides an empirical answer as to how the COVID-19 pandemic has transformed business relations and trust in business. Studying a wholesale market located in Paris (France), he shows how, at a time when social contacts are reduced to a minimum, social and personal relationships still shape market transactions.

Finally, the chapters by Li and Pang, Zhang and You and Faret et al. provide us with the perspective of how transnational communities negotiate trust within their own transnational communities and with the local communities where they are located in. On the basis of the ethnographic survey of a Chinese school in Belgium, Li and Pang look at Belgian immigrants' strategies and practices to adopt the Chinese approach to combat the pandemic in the Belgian context. They argue that immigrants sought to localize China's approach into the Belgian environment, transcending the binary choice between China and Belgium in coping and living with the coronavirus. Zhang and You explore another Chinese immigrant community in the American state of Florida. They argue that a trusted and efficient community-based organization is an essential force to unite and utilize local resources in trying times. Finally, the chapter by Faret et al. discusses how the pandemic is disrupting the systems of trust/distrust prevalent in the international corridor of Central America, Mexico and the United States. They argue that the pandemic contributes to the construction of figures suggesting danger and provoking fear, figures that are both institutional constructions and social representations of people on the move.

COVID-19 and its long tail

Two years after the first detection of the COVID-19 pandemic in 2019, this pandemic is still wrecking its toll on the global population with its various changing mutating variants. The tested COVID-19 vaccines and a huge vaccination program across the world, particularly in developed countries, where large segments of the population have been vaccinated with three doses of the mRNA COVID-19 vaccines and with the availability of COVID-19 oral drugs, there are still people being infected and reinfected. This is pegged against the backdrop of a shortage of vaccines in many developing countries where a large portion of the population remains unvaccinated. Strategies to cope with the spread of this highly transmissible infection ranged from whole city lockdown to herd immunity and now human–virus coexistence. For the first two years, countries throughout the world have adopted restricted border movements or closed their borders in the hope of stamping out this infection.

With a large segment of the world population having been vaccinated and the general effectiveness of the COVID-19 vaccines where those who were infected after being fully vaccinated (with two or three doses) suffering from non-life-threatening mild symptoms, governments in different countries have adopted a more relaxed approach to border opening. By early 2022, many countries had decided to adopt human–virus coexistence strategies and treat COVID-19 as an endemic, rather than the WHO-designated pandemic. With this strategy, countries are opening up their borders and allowing for the open but controlled movement of people and goods across continents and yet, at the same time, embracing the idea that the COVID-19 virus will continue to infect people in the community.

The key strategy and consideration in most countries is the management and governance of the local environment to ensure that the COVID-19 virus while living in the community is manageable through vaccines, oral medication and medical treatment. In this sense, through the transmission of medical knowledge and the availability of different methods of treatment, the global and local governments and scientific communities have sought to reduce the level of fear and risk and brought back scientific trust and trust in governance to the communities at the local and global levels.

In the final analysis, we learn COVID-19 and its long tail will continue to affect us but with the initial fear eliminated, people in different communities of the world will adapt and continue their familiar livelihood and lifestyle as they embraced this virus as part of the medical risks that are here to stay.

Notes

1 Khun Eng Kuah is the corresponding author.

2 "Wuhan Market was epicentre of pandemic's start: studies suggest". *Nature: News in Focus*. By Amy Maxmen, February 27, 2022. https://www.nature.com/articles/d41586-022-00584-8. Accessed March 8, 2022.

3 For detailed information, see "Covid-19 Coronavirus Pandemic". Worldometer. https://www.worldometers.info/coronavirus/. Accessed March 10, 2022.

4 For a country-to-country report on the daily COVID-19 infection rate, see Our World in Data. Oxford Martin School, University of Oxford. https://ourworldindata.org/search?q=covid+infection+. Accessed March 3, 2022.
5 For a discussion, see "Mask Diplomacy: Chinese Narratives in the COVID Era". *All FSI News/Blog*. Freeman Spogli Institute for International Studies, Stanford University. By Alicia Chen and Vanessa Molter, June 16, 2020. https://fsi.stanford.edu/news/covid-mask-diplomacy. Accessed March 8, 2022.
6 For a discussion on the various types of vaccines, see "The different types of Covid-19 vaccines". WHO, January 12, 2021. https://www.who.int/news-room/feature-stories/detail/the-race-for-a-covid-19-vaccine-explained?topicsurvey=v8kj13)&gclid=Cj0KCQiAmpyRBhC-ARIsABs2EAphMGop6hfYweHXv4tJ2tHCfeLxnSathWvsWlqQmTCRT3VFl1Ws3-4aAtIAEALw_wcB. Accessed March 9, 2022.
7 For details, see "Covid-19 vaccines". WHO. https://www.who.int/emergencies/diseases/novel-coronavirus-2019/covid-19-vaccines. Accessed March 9, 2022.
8 For details on the vaccination rate, see "Coronavirus (Covid-19) Vaccinations" Our World in Data. https://ourworldindata.org/covid-vaccinations. Accessed March 9, 2022.
9 For discussion of "herd immunity", see Coronavirus disease (COVID-19): Herd immunity, lockdowns and COVID-19. WHO, December 31, 2020. https://www.who.int/emergencies/diseases/novel-coronavirus-2019/question-and-answers-hub/q-a-detail/herd-immunity-lockdowns-and-covid-19?gclid=CjwKCAiAvaGRBhBlEiwAiY-yMOSGlywSPrQzPBO10SyKzoWuPEtjfL7yB8a5D3i7Z1EYndsu2imrKBoCZb0QAvD_BwE. Accessed March 10, 2022.
10 For details on this, see "Vaccine Inequality: Ensuring Africa is not left out". Brookings Foresight Africa Series. By Michel Sidibe. January 24, 2022. https://www.brookings.edu/blog/africa-in-focus/2022/01/24/vaccine-inequity-ensuring-africa-is-not-left-out/. Accessed March 10, 2022.
11 "New report reveals how food banks respond to COVID-19". Foodtank: The Think Tank for Food. August, 2021. https://foodtank.com/news/2021/08/new-report-reveals-how-food-banks-responded-to-covid/. Accessed March 10, 2022.

References

Anderson, B. 1983. *Imagined Communities: Reflections on the Origin and Spread of Nationalism*. London: Verso.

Barrios, R. E. 2014. "'Here, I'm not at ease': anthropological perspectives on community resilience". *Disasters*. 38 (2): 329–250. DOI: https://doi.org/10.1111/disa.12044.

Beck, U.1992. *Risk Society: Towards a New Modernity*. London: Sage.

Bell, C. and Newby, Hd. 1971. *Community Studies. An Introduction to the Sociology of the Local Community*. London: Allen and Unwin.

Bidard, C. and Lavenu D. 2005. "Evolutions of personal networks and life events". *Social Networks*. 27 (4): 359–376.

Bulmer, M. 1985. "The rejuvenation of community studies? Neighbour, networks and policy". *The Sociological Review*. 33 (3): 430–448.

Castells, M. 1968. "Y a-t-il une sociologie urbaine ?". *Sociologie du travail*. 10 (1): 72–90.

Charles, N. Aull Davies, C. 2005. "Studying the particular, illuminating the general: community studies and community in Wales". *The Sociological Review*. 53 (4): 672–690.

Cohen A. P., 1985, *Symbolic Construction of Community*, London: Routledge.

Frankenberg, R. 1966. *Communities in Britain: Social Life in Town and Country*. Harmondsworth: Penguin.

Frankenberg, R. 1990. *Village on the Border*. 2nd edition. Prospect Heights: Waveland Press.
Giddens, A. 1992. *The Transformation of Intimacy*. Stanford: Stanford University Press.
Putnam, R. 2000. *Bowling Alone: The Collapse and Revival of American Community*. New York: Simon and Schuste.
Stone, L. 1977. *The Family, Sex and Marriage in England 1500–1800*. London: Weidenfeld and Nicholson.
Tönnies, F. 1988. *Community and Society*. London: Routeledge.
Williams, R. 1973. *The Country and the City*. London: Chatto and Windus.

2 Trust and modalities of social action in the pandemic

Francis K. G. LIM

The COVID-19 pandemic has forced us to ask some difficult questions concerning the foundations of our social and political life. The SARS-CoV-2 virus has generated intense uncertainty and deep ambiguity in many aspects of social interactions that we had previously taken for granted. One of the most fundamental questions that arise is: who can be trusted to enter and inhabit our intimate or significant spaces such as the home, community and the nation? Relatedly, how can we conceptualize trust (and mistrust) when even our most significant social relations (such as parents, children and loved ones) are now feared because they may be infected and infectious, and hence to be spatially segregated through quarantine and "safe distancing" measures? At the same time, we also observe that certain groups (such as migrant workers and minorities) in society are experiencing heightened discrimination, physical violence and other forms of mistreatment because they are not trusted by the majority or powerful groups who positioned themselves as custodians of the wellbeing of the nation.

Since the COVID-19 outbreak, researchers have been studying the interactions between different kinds of trust and how individuals and societies perceive risk, implement restrictive measures and compliance. Devine et al. (2020) have provided a useful summary of this body of research. For example, higher political and societal trust in some European Union countries is linked to the late adoption of restrictive policies (Toshkov et al. 2020). Studies from the US and Denmark have shown that people with higher trust are more likely to comply with COVID-19 measures (Han et al. 2021; Olsen and Hjorth 2020). The caveat is that this may depend on who is issuing the orders. In the US, higher social trust seems to result in lower levels of compliance (Goldstein and Wiedemann 2020). Higher trust in government is associated with lower risk perception, while individuals with low trust in science and medical professionals tend to have higher risk perception (Dryhurst et al. 2020). In a survey of 28 countries, Edelman, a consultancy, has found that people's trust in their governments has fallen steeply in 2020, especially in the US and China (apnews.com). In addition, due to the spread of misinformation surrounding the vaccines, only around 30% of respondents indicate that they are willing to get a COVID-19 vaccine immediately. In Russia, for example, only 15% of those surveyed are willing to get vaccinated as soon as possible. In India, the figure is around 50%.

DOI: 10.4324/9781003291220-2

Studies cited in the previous paragraphs, as well as others, tend to utilize different theoretical approaches to examine how trust relates to issues of adoption of restrictive policies, compliance with such policies, risk perception, etc. This has resulted in findings that are difficult to compare across societies. For example, how can we explain findings that show higher trust with a higher likelihood of compliance, while higher social trust seems to result in lower levels of compliance? Also, given how trust, risk and blame are intertwined (Douglas 1994; Douglas and Wildavsky 1982), studies thus far have not adequately examined how different forms or levels of trust relate to blame. The pandemic has also given rise to many instances of verbal and physical attacks on minority communities and other marginalized groups in many countries. How is trust related to such incidents? Addressing the gap in the existing research, I propose the concept of *trust liminality* to analyze how the pandemic has resulted in a momentary suspension of trust in different contexts. Adapting the cultural theory approach developed by Mary Douglas and her collaborators, I then present a theoretical model comprising interactions of particularized and system trust that produce four modalities of social action. In analyzing how trust liminality is resolved, the model gives us insights into the interactions between trust, risk and blame in individuals and social groups. The model also provides a common analytical framework that can be used to compare different cases across societies and scales.

The chapter is organized as follows. I first briefly discuss the different approaches to trust and my use of particularized and system thrust to construct the model. This is followed by a detailed discussion of the concept of trust liminality and how it may be resolved with reference to legitimate authority. Next, I present the model of four modalities of social action and how it incorporates risk and blame in relation to the pandemic. Finally, I conclude with a summary of the key arguments.

Definitions of trust

Definitions of trust in the scholarly literature can be broadly categorized into either the functional or substantive definitions. My purpose here is not to provide an exhaustive review of the merits or inadequacies of all these available definitions (e.g., Misztal 1996; Hardin 2002; Hosking 2014; Frederiksen 2014). My aim here is to adopt a working definition for use in our subsequent analysis. A good example of a functional definition is provided by Luhmann. He conceptualizes trust as an act essential "for the reduction of a future characterized by more or less indeterminate complexity" and involves "the taking of a risk" (Luhmann 2017, 17, 79). For Luhmann, trust is not just a psychological coping mechanism but also a social action, with intersubjectivity as its basis (Frederiksen 2014; Kroeger 2019). Like trust, distrust also functions to reduce complexity. According to Luhmann, both trust and distrust involve generalizations. The former allows social actors to form positive expectations while the latter to form negative expectations.

> Anyone who does not trust must, therefore, turn to functionally equivalent strategies for the reduction of complexity in order to be able to define a

> practically meaningful situation at all. He must hone his expectations into negative ones, and so must, in certain respects, become distrustful.
>
> (Luhmann 2017, 79)

In contrast, Newton adopts a substantive definition of trust: it is "the belief that others will not deliberately or knowingly do us harm, if they can avoid it, and will look after our interests, if this is possible" (Newton 2007, 343). In combining both functional and substantive approaches for a more comprehensive definition, I define trust as a risk-taking act that reduces life's future complexity, based on the belief that others will not deliberately or knowingly do us harm and will look after our interests.

Trust is a broad concept that can be further distinguished into different types of trust. First, there is particularized trust or social trust, usually found in communities or groups with strong social bonds underpinned by common values, interests or worldviews. This kind of trust comprises like-minded people who interact closely with and are dependent upon one another (Williams 1988; Newton 2007). Ideally, these closely bonded groups tend to have a relatively homogenous culture with powerful social sanctions. Members are socialized into a common culture and strive to forge a strong in-group identity. For members of such groups, legitimate authority lies in individuals or entities that are seen as best embodying the values, norms and worldview of the group. While group members tend to trust one another, they are less trustful of people in the out-groups (Gambetta 1988; cf. Douglas and Wildavsky 1982, on sectarian groups).

The other kind of trust that concerns us here is system trust, where social systems (e.g., political, medical, technological, economic) are the objects of trust. This entails that the trustor "assumes that a system is functioning and places his trust in that function and not in … people" (Luhmann 2017, 55). Typically, characteristics of system trust include independence from individual motivation (e.g., trust in money) and the requirement of expert knowledge to exercise control over it. System trust exists in a complex relationship with particularized, interpersonal trust and can both substitute and complement each other (Kroeger 2019, 166). As Luhmann (2017, 58) asks, "Does one trust the chemist, or his assistant, or the doctor, or is it medicine, science or technology?"

All social actors are simultaneously embedded within both personal networks and systems. To varying degrees, both shape people's meaning-making efforts and their social actions. Examples of personal networks are those of the immediate family and wider kin groups, intimate acquaintances, friends, religious or spiritual communities, voluntary associations, interest groups and political parties. At the same time, individuals and their social networks are embedded within systems that are ideal typically underpinned by impersonal rules and norms, highly abstract and technical knowledge or formal rationality. Such systems include the political and economic systems, highly specialized professions and state bureaucracies.

The pandemic has shattered the familiar world that is the precondition for trust (Luhmann 2017, 22). People have been jolted into stark realization that the world is socially contingent and compelled to engage in the construction of new meanings. I propose the concept of trust liminality to describe the rupture of the familiar world and hence the temporary suspension of trust and distrust in both personal networks and wider systems.

Trust liminality

> Familiarity is the precondition for trust as well as distrust, i.e., for every sort of commitment to a particular attitude towards the future ... The past does not contain any "other possibilities"; complexity is reduced at the outset. Thus an orientation to things past can simplify the world and render it less harmful.
>
> (Luhmann 2017, 22, 23)

Trust liminality refers to the temporary suspension of both particularized trust (in close groups) and system trust (e.g., in science, government, technology, etc.). My use of the term "liminality" is drawn from the work of Arnold van Gennep (1903) and Victor Turner (1964). For van Gennep, liminality refers to a transitional period in rites of passage. Turner uses the concept in his study of the Ndembu to describe a "betwixt and between" in coming-of-age rituals whereby participants shed their old identity but have not yet assumed a new one. Here, trust liminality refers to situations in which individuals or social groups are confronted by a *new* situation that compels them to decide whether, what or whom to trust or distrust so that they can engage in subsequent social actions. Following Turner's characterization of liminality, trust liminality is a leveling condition whereby everyone is neither trusted nor distrusted.

During the pandemic, trust liminality has proliferated in all domains of social life. Because of the unprecedented nature of the coronavirus, many existing social and behavioral norms, medical expertise, technical knowledge and modes of governance are unable to adequately deal with its widespread impacts. At the same time, societies are still struggling to formulate and agree upon the appropriate social norms to handle the pandemic while finding the technical knowledge to curb the spread of the virus. In a "betwixt and between" stage of "pre-COVID" and "post-COVID", societies around the world are in a liminal or transitional state where the foundations of trust are questioned, negotiated, contested or reformulated as individuals and social groups decide on the appropriate actions to take in their everyday life.

For particularized trust, individuals constantly face situations where they have to deal with questions of whether or not to trust other social actors in close-knit groups. If parents wished to visit their children during a lockdown while downplaying the risks and declared themselves to be well, should their children agree? Should mass religious services be held when such events might increase the risk of viral transmission? Should a father kiss his baby after coming home from work as a public transport worker?

For system trust, individuals and social groups face situations in which they ask if they should trust political leaders, public health officials, the police, medical experts, scientists and other public authorities on the appropriate actions to take. For example, in the domain of medical science, trust liminality can consist of people questioning the safety and efficacy of the new vaccines. New medical breakthroughs need to be thoroughly tested, new protocols formulated and new rules governing vaccine distribution devised. Meanwhile, past knowledges and social norms may be inadequate to deal with the pandemic and its impacts on society. In line with the definition of trust in this chapter, for individuals and social groups momentarily experiencing system trust liminality, future complexities are not reduced by existing expert systems to guide social actions. Concomitantly, there is an urgent re-assessment of the risks associated with COVID-19 and who or what may potentially be the sources of harm.

For both particularized and system trust liminality, a key point to note is that the condition of liminality cannot remain unresolved for an extended period. Both types of liminality are a momentary pause. Individuals and social groups need to move into a post-liminal state to engage in future acts. Imagine the following scenario: someone is about the enter a building when she sees a notice that informing those entering the premise to scan a QR code using their mobile phones to check-in and to allow contact tracing by the government health authority should the need arises. *How* she would act, I would argue, depends crucially on the legitimate authority or authorities she appeals to, *viz.* an authority within her closely bonded group or systemic authority, or both. In this sense, trust liminality conceptually differs from Möllering's (2001) notion of trust suspension, which compels the actor to make a "leap of faith" in order to trust. While trust liminality also involves a condition of suspension, the subsequent social action undertaken is not so much dependent on faith as on attribution of authority, a process I term *trust enactment*: this is the resolution of trust liminality resulting from one's conferring of trust on persons and/or systems whose authority is deemed legitimate. In other words, the decision on what is the appropriate action to take in the transition to a post-liminal state depends crucially on what or who social actors consider as legitimate authority (hence *trustworthy*).

To reiterate: in any social context, individuals and social groups are embedded within particularized and system trust to varying degrees. The strengths of these two forms of trust may be correlated either positively or inversely relative to each other, but none is completely absent. Therefore, social actions may be conceptualized as resulting from the dynamic interplay between particularized and system trust. An individual may act due to their higher particularized trust relative to system trust, or vice versa. There could be situations that social actions are derived from one type of trust and the distrust of the other. For instance, an "anti-vaxxer" may adamantly refuse to be administered COVID vaccine (as a social action) because they trust their close friend's negative opinions on vaccination while distrusting the government's words on vaccine safety and efficacy. Trust liminality can also be resolved when individuals engage in social actions based on their trust in *both* close personal networks and the system.

Modalities of social action: a conceptual framework

Based on the interactions between system trust and particularized trust, I propose four possible modalities of social action or trust enactment engaged in by individuals and social groups. These modalities are analytically distinct but one or more may be empirically present in any particular social groups or individuals (cf. Fardon 2013, 54). Empirically, any individual or social group may grapple with several modalities in a contested ranking in a single instance of trust liminality. Any individual, as a social being, is at the same time embedded temporally and spatially. As an individual moves through the course of a day, they may encounter many instances of trust liminality in different contexts that may result in different trust enactments. In relation to authority, these different contexts may present a different hierarchy or configuration of authority to the individual. Their choices of the appropriate course of action will hence be shaped by the dynamic interactions of system and social trust in these specific contexts and times.

Risk and blame in modalities of social action

Following Douglas's ([1966] 2004) characterization of "dirt" as "matter out of place", I suggest that it is analytically useful to consider SARS-CoV-2 as a kind of polluting, formless dirt. For Douglas, dirt comprises anomalous elements that do not 'fit' into pre-existing social order, and the idea of dirt is related to societal concerns with contagion. In this sense, the emergence of SARS-CoV-2 as "COVID dirt" can be regarded as the irruption of a new anomalous entity in human society, confounding the expertise of the scientists and medical experts, posing severe and deadly threats to people's health, and disrupting existing social relations. Individuals, social groups and societies are still finding ways to deal with the coronavirus medically, politically, societally and economically. Our model thus provides a theoretical framework to analyze how individuals and groups deal with the COVID dirt with respect to whom or what they trust, as they search for appropriate actions in response to COVID-19 outbreak.

Each of the modalities in our theoretical model presupposes its distinct cultural framing of risk induced by the COVID dirt, and assigns blame based on the framing. Douglas and Wildavsky (1982) argue that risk assessment is not empirically given but is interpreted within a cultural frame. Regarding environmental risk in the US, for example, Douglas and Wildasky show that for some of the more extreme environmental groups, there was "a single, overriding societal threat in order to support their own survival as voluntary organizations", and that they use this threat "simultaneously to hold their membership together and to attack the hierarchies they oppose". Criticizing the risk consultancy industry in perpetuating the myth of risk assessment as a purely technical matter and couching it in a veneer of objectivity, Douglas and Wildavsky argue that a society is never so settled or certain of its values that "its processes for discovering the facts and making political decisions would be judged fully adequate", and that there is usually no agreement "over appropriate methods to assess risks nor acceptance of the outcomes of public processes" (Douglas and Wildavsky 1982, 68). Fundamentally, that which is considered risky is not something that exists objectively "out there", completely dissociated from human subjectivity. On the contrary, risk assessment is biased and very much a matter of judgment that is formed with reference to shared beliefs and values (ibid., 194). Applying this cultural approach of risk assessment to COVID dirt in our theoretical model, each of the four modalities of social action is associated with its analytically distinct cultural framing of risk deriving from the relative levels of system and particularized trust.

This brings us to the related issue of blame. For Douglas, the category of risk is integral to a society's blaming system. For example, if on the one side is the identification of environmental risk, on the other lies the object of blame, e.g., big corporations. The targets of accusation will first attract libel as the main culprits for the presence of socially threatening, anomalous elements. They will be imputed with alleged moral weakness for degradation, acquiring the status of "dirt" that needs to be impugned from society through preventive actions (Douglas 1992, 85–88). A sociological model of the risks posed by infectious diseases such as COVID-19 will involve not only examining their virological and epidemiological aspects, but also how society at large constructs the objects of blame as the sources of risk and therefore threats to its order and moral values. In relation to the substantive issue of trust, the blame targets are socially constructed as "high risk" and therefore cannot be trusted.

Following from the above discussions, I propose the theoretical model comprising four modalities of social actions for the resolution of trust liminality in the pandemic. I elaborate on each modality in the following paragraphs.

Synchronized modality

The synchronized modality comprises social actions that result from the resolution of trust liminality as a function of high legitimacy attributed to both system trust and particularized trust. In this modality individuals from close-knit social groupings would generally confer legitimacy on broader systems and their representatives regarding appropriate actions to deal with various aspects of the pandemic. For example, ethnic and religious communities, civic groups or professional organizations may collaborate with doctors, scientists, public health officials and lawmakers to plan and execute common responses to the pandemic. This modality can be the outcome of the presence of both high political and social trust. For example, a religious group may exhort its members to follow strictly the government guidelines on the protocols for safe distancing, testing and contact tracing, and put in place COVID safety measures at the sites for religious activities. This is because group members confer high levels of legitimacy on both religious (particularized trust) and public authorities (system trust).

Regarding risk and blame, since individuals and social groups consider both system and close social networks as legitimate authority, there is a general convergence of views over the identification of risks and their sources as well as the targets of blame. For example, individuals and social groups may mostly agree with the views of experts such as virologists, epidemiologists, doctors and public health authorities on the health risks posed by the SARS-CoV-2 virus and how it is transmitted. The experts, on their part, could generally rely on social groups or

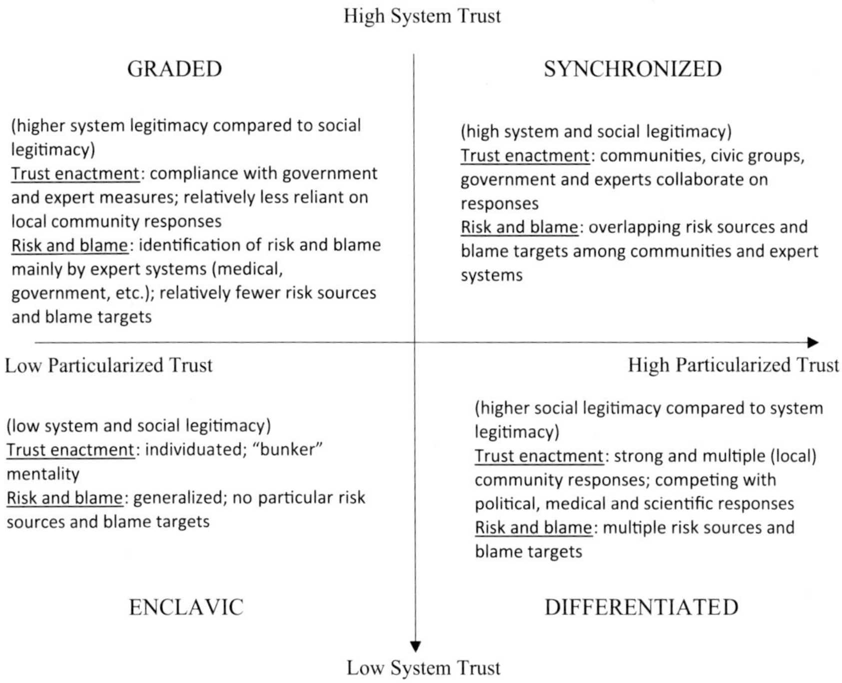

Figure 2.1 A model of social action in the pandemic.

individuals to adhere to the public guidelines on appropriate behaviors to mitigate the risks. Meanwhile, at the societal level, a strong consensus may prevail on who or what are the sources of risks and hence to blame and sanctioned for COVID-related threats. Sanctions against these blame targets will be sustained and severe since contrarian opinions may be few or weak. In terms of identity politics, there may be strong "Othering" processes that construct clear, distinct in-group boundaries against an out-group that are synonymous with COVID threats. Such an "Other" is imputed with moral failings, regarded with intense fear or loathing and therefore distrusted.

Differentiated modality

The differentiated modality is characterized by high levels of particularized trust competing with or eclipsing system trust. That is, individuals and social groups place as much, or more, trust in their close-knit social networks than in the wider expert systems such as the pharmaceutical industry and public health authorities. In this modality, there can be multiple, varied and assertive community and localized responses to the pandemic, competing and contrasting with political, medical or scientific responses. In other words, there is no society-wide consensus on the appropriate measures to deal with the pandemic. For example, individuals or groups may question the experts' views on the origins, health dangers and other negative effects of the virus while putting forth alternative theories and opinions. This could result in groups of experts and their critics dismissing each other's views as "fake news" or "conspiracy theories". For example, Goldstein and Weidemann (2020) have found that social or particularized trust is negatively correlated with compliance, thus highlighting the factor of partisanship. In Germany, there were protests against anti-coronavirus public health measures (DW.com, February 15, 2021). Many protestors were part of a growing movement called the Querdenker ("lateral thinkers"), an alliance of mainly far-right and far-left groups and a few "conspiracy theorists". The Querdenker protestors claimed to support the fundamental right of freedoms of opinion, expression and assembly as enshrined in the German Basic Law. They were united in their distrust of mainstream information on the virus and government measures to deal with the pandemic. In August 2020, some Querdenker protestors in Berlin tried unsuccessfully to barge into the parliament building.

In a differentiated modality, we can expect contentions over the identifications of risk and measures of risk mitigation, and multiple objects of blame. In a way, this may be a function of a relatively assertive and autonomous civil society *vis-à-vis* the state. In countries where citizens display relatively low trust in their governments and public institutions, when the latter are deemed incompetent in dealing with the pandemic-induced health, economic, political or social crises, civil society groups (e.g., voluntary welfare organizations, professional groups, religious institutions, ethnic or local communities) may seek solutions on their own or through collaborating with one another.

There can be two potential outcomes from such social actions. One, civil society groups in their respective efforts may result in positive social outcomes by providing much-needed services to deal with the pandemic which the public authorities are unable to deliver. On the other hand, multifarious, uncoordinated or even competing approaches by civil society groups can result in disagreements over the proper channeling of resources and intractable disputes over the appropriate responses to the pandemic. This may further undermine trust in public institutions and other systems. For example, compared with the rest of the world, France had one of the highest levels of "vaccine hesitancy", with many French people unwilling to get inoculated. The main reason was apparently a deep distrust of government and the experts. Past government mishandlings of vaccination efforts, such as the backtracking of the rollout of hepatitis B vaccine in 1994 and a massive over purchase of H1N1 swine flu vaccine in 2009, have contributed to the French public's distrust of policymakers (*The Guardian*, February 15, 2021).

In their chapter on the COVID responses of displaced slum dwellers in Delhi, Dupont and Shankare discuss the prominent role played by community-based organizations and NGOs in helping slum dwellers deal with multiple risks associated with the pandemic. Many residents looked to their old and new local community organizations and NGOs more than state institutions in seeking assistance with their problems. As an example of differentiated modality, the slum dwellers' trust enactment involved different kinds of organizations, state and non-state, with many placing their trust in their own close social networks more than in the government. Like the Querdenker movement in Germany, this case study shows how high levels of particularized or social trust can compete with or eclipsing system trust (especially political trust).

Because individuals and social groups may adopt different interpretive frames, bodies of knowledge, ideologies or worldviews in dealing with various aspects of the pandemic, they also may identify different risk sources and blame targets. In other words, in a differentiated modality, there can be a multiplicity of risk interpretations and responses as well as objects of blame. For example, since the COVID outbreak in early 2020, there have been reports of rising attacks against Asians or citizens of Asian descent in the US and some European countries. The Asian American Bar Association of New York reports that from January to November 2020, anti-Asian hate crimes handled by the New York Police Department spiked 800% compared to the same period in 2019. Commentators have attributed this sharp rise in verbal and physical attacks on ethnic Asians partly to the view among certain groups that COVID-19 was a "China virus", a view promoted by the former US president, Donald Trump. Responding within the political system, President Joe Biden said that the "inflammatory and xenophobic rhetoric has put Asian American and Pacific Islander (AAPI) persons, families, communities, and businesses at risk". He then ordered the Department of Health and Human Services "to consider issuing Covid-19 guidance to address issues to language access and sensitivity toward the AAPI community" (CNN).

Scientists, medical experts, health officials and lawmakers, as system representatives, may strive to provide biomedical and virological explanations for the origins and spread of the Sars-CoV-2. They may also seek to curb xenophobia and hate crimes against certain ethnic groups. In a differentiated modality, as in the US as previously mentioned, a considerable number of individuals and social groups may not confer high levels of legitimacy on such experts or politicians and are distrustful of their efforts. Therefore, the differentiated modality offers a plausible explanation for the spike in cases of racially motivated hate crimes around the world during the pandemic. Individuals and groups may have a relatively higher particularized trust compared to system trust and hence more accepting of the alternative views promulgated by their own close networks, including views that certain social groups or nationalities are to blame for the pandemic.

Graded modality

The graded modality is characterized by higher system legitimacy compared to social legitimacy. That is, *in relative terms*, individuals or groups trust systems more than their close social circles. This means that when there are divergences of opinions over the appropriate actions to take in response to the pandemic, individuals and social groups will generally seek guidance from expert systems and public institutions due to their perceived higher legitimacy. An important question is: in a context of high levels of system trust, how will individuals or the public, in general, behave in response to the COVID advisories of the government authorities and/or experts?

On the one hand, some recent studies on the COVID-19 pandemic have found that, in line with past research, higher trust in government results in higher citizen compliance with restrictive measures such as quarantine, social distancing and testing (e.g., Han et al. 2021; Olsen and Hjorth 2020). On the other hand, there are also other studies that provide a contrasting picture, where higher trust in government, as a form of system trust, may have the opposite effect of *lower compliance* as individuals may feel a decreased sense of personal responsibility and urgency in adhering to the containment measures. For example, Wong and Jensen (2020) have studied the interaction between trust in government, risk perceptions and public compliance in Singapore, where public trust in government is high compared to other high-income countries. Through social media tracking and focus group interviews, the authors' preliminary findings suggest that the high level of trust in the Singaporean government among the study respondents (comprising Singaporeans and non-Singaporeans) seems to be correlated with the low levels of perceived risk, resulting in low compliance with the government's COVID measures. To generalize, the study's main findings indicate the possibility that in a graded modality, higher levels of system trust (in government and other expert systems) may, in some instances, result in a lower sense of individual responsibility or ability to manage risks.

We may also ask whether the high levels of compliance observed are due to higher trust placed on systems, or more to threats of sanctions on non-compliance imposed by state authorities. In other words, could compliance be due to fear rather than trust? It is certainly plausible that people may comply with restrictive measures due to their fear of government sanctions. For example, if the flouting of laws forbidding certain activities could potentially land a person in jail, that person's compliance with such laws may not be due to trust in public authorities so much as fear of legal sanctions. This is especially likely in politically authoritarian states where there is as much rule by fear as rule of law, where political dissensions are often met with harsh responses by the authorities. Empirically, therefore, similar behavioral outcomes may be seen in situations of graded modality (where there is high system or public trust relative to particularized trust) and situations where coercion or force is more a factor than trust in people's compliance with COVID response measures.

Our model suggests that, under the graded modality, the identification of risk and blame is likely to be system-led. For example, public authorities and experts in specialized fields may dominate the discourse on important aspects of the pandemic and are the main shapers of the responses to the pandemic. Various branches of the government may work closely with medical professionals, scientists and other health experts in devising policy responses to the pandemic in areas such as public health, the economy, social activities, education, vaccine development and inoculation. They publicly identify the groups and activities which pose the most risk to public health. As a result, system representatives construct in the public sphere the potential blame targets, such as when they identify groups or individuals flouting the pandemic curbing measures. Such "high-risk" groups are identified and "shamed" by the authorities, the media institutions and the public's use of various media platforms (e.g., social media). Publicly stigmatized and marginalized at the broad societal level, such groups may experience sanctions as forms of punishment.

On the issue of power, the overwhelming system of authority comprising state bureaucracies, public institutions and expert groups makes it very difficult for the targeted groups to counter the negative narratives and sanctions directed at them. For example, the accepted view around the world concerning the origins of the Sars-CoV-2 is that it first emerged in China, possibly through transmission from bats into the human food chain via the sale and consumption of wildlife meats in the country. The pandemic appears to have started in the city of Wuhan or the surrounding areas, resulting in the labeling of COVID-19 by some as a "Chinese virus". In order to counteract the world's negative image of China concerning the origins and rapid spread of the virus (due to alleged initial government missteps), as well as to deflect the blame, the Chinese government and the country's official media outlets have been pushing an alternative theory that the virus had entered China from overseas through imported frozen foods. In other words, in China, the dominant political narrative in the public media constructs that Sars-Cov-2 as a "foreign" virus. Alternative interpretations and voices are hence either marginalized or suppressed in the country.

Enclavic modality

The enclavic modality is associated with conditions of low system trust and low social trust. In terms of trust enactment, people engaging in this modality attribute low legitimacy to both system experts and social networks, resulting in highly individualized responses. They may feel a strong sense of generalized, existential crisis relating to aspects of the human condition such as global environmental calamity, threats of nuclear disasters and deadly pandemics. Because they consider the root causes of such threats to humanity as largely systemic (e.g., problems of socio-technical systems, global geopolitics, governance, modernization, consumerism, etc.), they eschew looking to broad expert systems for solutions to humanity's existential challenges. At the same time, these individuals are not deeply embedded in social networks and do not regard particularized social groupings as able to provide solutions to the generalized threats they face. In terms of political orientation, they tend to be attracted to libertarian ideals and values such as individual freedom, autonomy, self-reliance and laissez-faire economics and politics.

An example of enclavic modality is provided by Garrett's (2021) study of the doomsday "preppers" around the world. The preppers are preparing for conditions of calamity "which they believe inevitable and have been exponentially escalated through human hubris and excessive reliance on technology and global trade networks" (Garrett 2021). For example, in Kansas, US, a property developer acquired a former government bunker and rebuilt it into a 15-story underground tower block, the Survival Condo. The luxurious facility allows residents to survive for five years following cataclysmic events and is equipped with nuclear, biological, water and chemical air filtration units. Survival Condo's website claimed that its filtration systems were able to screen out the COVID-19 virus.

It is important to note that those engaging in enclavic modality do not necessarily distrust expert systems or social groups as such. For example, the preppers do trust expert knowledge and technical systems to build and maintain their ultra-secure bunkers to keep them safe. Many of these preppers would also want to move into the bunkers with their close social groups, such as their families or other preppers. The sense of distrust among those in enclavic modality is more generalized, and not directed at specific systems or social groups. It is based on judgments concerning some trends or developments of human society or the environment, such as global militarization, the proliferation of nuclear technology, global environmental degradation and climate change, deadly epidemics or other "ills" of modernity.

This means that in enclavic modality, risk and blame take on a more generalized nature. With reference to the COVID pandemic, for example, the attribution of blame is directed less at specific groups or individuals and more at how humanity as a whole organizes and sustains itself through the exploitation of natural resources, rampant capitalism, unrestrained consumerism, antagonistic relations and so on. Individuals or social groups may be blamed only in so far as they are regarded as representatives or agents of broader industries, activities, systems or social organizations that underlie the generalized risks and threats. For example, rather than the racist overtones in the attribution of blame for the COVID pandemic among some groups in other modalities (e.g., Sars-CoV-2 as a "Chinese virus"), those in the enclavic modality would more likely direct their criticisms and displeasure at the prevailing system of food production and consumption, as well as governments' regulatory regimes.

Conclusion

As it sweeps across the globe, the Sars-CoV-2 virus has been threatening and disruptive on many fronts. Due to the many new uncertainties and complexities that have emerged from the pandemic, individuals, social groups and nations are faced with situations where much of the erstwhile norms, rules and knowledges that have previously guided behaviors and policies are found to be inadequate or in need of a drastic overhaul. With the emergence of a new coronavirus, past experiences no longer could serve as a reliable guide for individuals and societies on the appropriate actions to take. If, following Luhmann, trust and distrust are the reduction of indeterminate complexities and the simplifying of risks to enable social action, the new complexities and risks resulting from the initial outbreak of the COVID-19 pandemic would have presented many individuals and social groups with situations whereby they have to decide on whom and what to trust so that the new complexities can be reduced and new risks managed. I have proposed the concept of trust liminality to describe the temporary suspension of trust in the pandemic. To resolve trust liminality, social actors reference the legitimate authorities in their social networks (particularized trust) and/or wider systems (system trust) to decide on the appropriate actions (trust enactment). A model of four types of social action is proposed to explain how trust liminality is handled as a function of the interactions between particularized trust and system trust. Crucially, the model also allows us to examine how each modality deals with risk and blame.

Individuals and social groups may experience trust liminality in all sorts of contexts (personal, group, nation, etc.) and domains (social, economic, political), and across different scales (micro, meso or macro). For example, at the personal level, one may be compelled to deliberate over the choice of one or more modalities in face of trust liminality. Should I visit my elderly parents regularly when I am not infected, when they express a strong desire to see me? Should I trust my parents' judgment that it is fine for me to visit them, or my own assessment of the situation, or should I trust the experts? Should my religious congregation continue to meet regularly for worship even with high rates of infection in society, because for us religion in the most important thing in life? Or should we adhere to government guidelines on social distancing and avoid gathering in large groups? Should I just confine myself to my home, stock up on months of food supply and other necessities and avoid most social contact? At a societal level, different civic, religious, and political groups may agree or disagree among themselves on who is to be trusted on matters such as the origins of the virus, who or what embodies "high risk", the appropriate responses to take to contain the pandemic, and the apportioning of blame. The model of four modalities enables us to understand and explain how trust liminality may be handled by individuals and social groupings across these diverse contexts and scales.

One of the greatest challenges for many governments to deal effectively with the pandemic is to convince their citizens to adhere to certain behavioral rules (e.g., social distancing, use of contract tracing apps), personal health measures (e.g., wearing face masks, using hand sanitizers) and public health initiatives (e.g., lockdown measures, vaccination). Among certain individuals and groups, there are high levels of mistrust of advisories and information provided by governmental, medical and scientific authorities. Added to this are the so-called "fake news" and "conspiracy theories", and misinformation circulating on different social media platforms. With reference to our theoretical model, various authorities (as representatives of "systems") may have limited success in embarking on educational and information campaigns to change the minds of these groups of critics, doubters and believers of "fake news". This is because, for many of these individuals and groups, their trust enactment rests more on their adherence to the legitimate authority within their own particularized social groups and less on the supposed "expertise" of health and governmental authorities. For example, to persuade vaccine doubters to get inoculated, it may be a more effective strategy for government health officials to identify the source of legitimate authority within the particularized group to which these doubters belong, and try to convince and work with this authoritative source as an essential step at persuasion.

Anthony Fauci, the director of the National Institute of Allergy and Infectious Diseases, was asked in a news program about a poll that found Republican men and Donald Trump supporters had the highest rates of vaccine hesitancy. Fauci said that "it makes absolutely no sense" to him that "such a large proportion of a certain group of people would not want to get vaccinated merely because of political consideration". For Fauci, getting vaccinated was a "common-sense, no-brainer public health thing" (*The Washington Post*, March 22, 2021). That which makes "no sense" to Fauci and other health officials can in fact be explained in terms of differentiated modality in our theoretical model. For those Republican men and Trump supporters who distrusted the vaccines, the source of legitimate authority that was the basis of trust enactment in an unprecedented event, rested less in the expert systems than in their respective strongly bonded political groupings. While Fauci may have professed a lack of understanding of the doubters' strong vaccine hesitation, he unwittingly stumbled upon the solution that is in line with what our theoretical model would suggest. Speaking on another TV channel, Fauci suggested that Donald Trump should encourage his supporters to get inoculated, since the former US president was still "a very widely popular person among Republicans" and that any push by him "would make all the difference in the world" (ibid.).

While the model delineates four distinct modalities, they should be considered ideal types that are being distinguished for analytical purposes. In any given real life situation of trust liminality confronting individuals, social groups or societies, one or more of the four modalities may be present and jostling for dominance. In individuals and within social groups, this may take the form of intense deliberations, raging doubts, internal quarrels and searching for more authoritative guidance or assurance. At the societal level, the attempts at seeking a resolution to trust liminality may involve broader political processes of contestations between public authorities and civil society groups. These processes can be relatively civil or take on more malicious forms such as physical attacks, violent protest movements and state suppression. Therefore, empirically the proposed model alerts us to the likelihood of what Douglas calls "culture clashes" in matters of compliance, risk assessment and apportioning of blame.

It also needs to be highlighted that the model is not a static framework. Luhmann correctly points out, as aligns with my view, that factors of time and information need to be part of any discussion on trust and trustworthiness. Individuals, social groups and societies are embedded in changing time and space, and this means that following a particular trust enactment, contexts may change when new, additional information becomes available to social actors over time. The change in contexts may prompt re-evaluations of the sources of legitimate authority, potentially resulting in social actors engaging a new modality.

Finally, the proposed model is useful for both explanatory and predictive purposes. It also provides a coherent theoretical framework and conceptual vocabulary for the comparative analysis of different cases and scenarios. As an explanatory model, it helps us understand what may be empirically observed in the behavioral patterns of individuals and social groups with respect to trust.

For example, we can compare and explain different individuals' refusal or willingness to get inoculated in relation to the relative extent to which they trust their respective close social networks *vis-à-vis* particular expert systems. On a more macro scale, the seemingly contested or chaotic responses to deal with the pandemic in a particular society can now be explained with greater conceptual clarity and coherence with reference to differentiated modality. The model also allows us to compare across societies, so that the different situations concerning compliance, risk assessment and blame can be explained from the perspective of a single explanatory framework. For predictive purposes, the model allows us to generate hypotheses. For example, we can use survey data on levels of system trust and particularized trust as independent variables and formulate hypotheses regarding how individuals or groups within and across societies may respond to various COVID-19 curbing measures. At the same time, we can also hypothesize about how these individuals and groups make risk assessments and attribute blame.

References

Devine, D., J. Gaskell, W. Jennings, and G. Stoker. 2020. "Trust and the Coronavirus Pandemic: What are the Consequences of and for Trust? An Early Review of the Literature." *Political Studies Review* 19 (2): 1–12. doi: 10.1177/1478929920948684.

Douglas, Mary. 1994. *Risk and Blame*. London: Routledge.

Douglas, Mary. 2004 [1966]. *Purity and Danger*. London: Routledge.

Douglas, Mary, and Aaron Wildavsky. 1982. *Risk and Culture: An Essay on the Selection of Technological and Environmental Dangers*. Berkeley: University of California Press.

Dryhurst, S., C.R. Schneider, J. Kerr, et al. 2020. "Risk Perceptions of COVID-19 Around the World." *Journal of Risk Research* 23: 7–8, 994–1006. doi: 10.1080/13669877.2020.1758193.

DW. 2021. "Coronavirus: Germany Braces for Anti-lockdown Protests." Accessed 15 February 2021. https://www.dw.com/en/coronavirus-germany-braces-for-anti-lockdown-protests/a-55513848

Fardon, Richard, ed. 2013. *Mary Douglas: Cultures and Crises*. London: Sage.

Frederiksen, Morten. 2014. "Trust in the Face of Uncertainty: A Qualitative Study of Intersubjective Trust and Risk." *International Review of Sociology* 24 (1): 130–144. doi: 10.1080/03906701.2014.894335.

Gambetta, Diego. 1988. "Can we Trust Trust?" In *Trust*, edited by D. Gambetta, 213–237. Oxford: Blackwell.

Garret, B. 2021. "Doomsday Preppers and the Architecture of Dread." *Geoforum* 127: 401–411.

Goldstein, D. and J. Wiedemann. 2020. "Who Do You Trust? The Consequences of Political and Social Trust for Public Responsiveness to COVID-19 Orders." http://dx.doi.org/10.2139/ssrn.3580547.

Han, Q., Zheng, B., Cristea, M., Agostini, M., Bélanger, J., Gützkow, B., et al. 2021. "Trust in Government Regarding COVID-19 and Its Associations with Preventive Health Behaviour and Prosocial Behaviour During the Pandemic: A Cross-Sectional and Longitudinal Study." *Psychological Medicine*: 1–11. doi:10.1017/S0033291721001306.

Hardin, Russell. 2002. *Trust and Trustworthiness*. New York: Sage.

Hosking, Geoffrey. 2014. *Trust: A History*. Oxford: Oxford University Press.

Kaur, Harmeet. 2021. "As Attacks Against Asian Americans Spike, Advocates Call for Action to Protect Communities." *CNN Report*, February 13. Accessed 13 February 2021. https://edition.cnn.com/2021/02/13/us/asian-american-attacks-COVID-19-hate-trnd/index.html

Kroeger, Frens. 2019. "Unlocking the Treasure Trove: How can Luhmann's Theory of Trust Enrich Trust Research?" *Journal of Trust Research* 9 (1): 110–124. doi: 10.1080/21515581.2018.1552592.

Luhmann, Niklas. 2017. *Trust and Power*. Cambridge: Polity.

Misztal, Barbara A. 1996. *Trust in Modern Societies*. Cambridge: Polity.

Möllering, Guido. 2001. "The Nature of Trust: From Georg Simmel to a Theory of Expectation, Interpretation and Suspension." *Sociology* 35 (2): 403–420.

Newton, Kenneth. 2007. "Social and Political Trust." In *The Oxford Handbook of Political Behaviour*, edited by R.J. Dalton, 343–361. Oxford: Oxford University Press.

Olsen, A.L. and F. Hjorth. 2020. "Willingness to Distance in the COVID-19." *OSF Preprints*. Available at: https:// osf.io/xpwg2/

Pylas, Pan. 2021. "Survey Finds Global Mistrust Could Weigh on Vaccine Rollout." *Associated Press*, January 13. Accessed 15 February 2021. https://apnews.com/article/coronavirus-pandemic-coronavirus-vaccine-united-states-3a6fbf0e8ff3e63917f707aa935b492c.

Toshkov, D., B. Caroll and K. Yesilkagit. 2020. "Government Capacity, Societal Trust or Party Preferences: What Accounts for the Variety of National Policy Responses to the COVID-19 Pandemic in Europe?" *Journal of European Public Policy* 29 (7): 1009–1028. doi: 10.1080/13501763.2021.1928270.

Turner, Victor. 1964. "Betwixt and Between: The Liminal Period in *Rites de Passage*." *The Proceedings of the American Ethnological Society*: 4–20.

Van Gennep, A. 1960. *The Rites of Passage*. Chicago: University of Chicago Press.

Wang, Amy B. 2021. "Fauci Says Trump Should Push Supporters To Get COVID Vaccine After 'Disturbing' Poll Results Show They Won't." *Washington Post*, 2021. Accessed 22 March 2021. https://www.washingtonpost.com/nation/2021/03/14/fauci-trump-supporters-vaccine/

Williams, Bernard. 1988. "Formal Structures and Social Reality." In *Trust: Making and Breaking Cooperative Relations*, edited by D. Gambetta, 3–15. Oxford: Blackwell.

Wong, C. M. L., and O. Jensen. 2020. "The Paradox of Trust: Perceived Risk and Public Compliance During the COVID-19 Pandemic in Singapore." *Journal of Risk Research* 23 (7–8): 1021–1030. doi: 10.1080/13669877.2020.1756386.

3 Practicing safe eating during the COVID-19 pandemic in Hong Kong

A trust in action perspective

Chong Gao and Khun Eng Kuah[1]

Introduction

COVID-19 is an acute respiratory illness caused by a newly identified coronavirus (SARS-CoV-2) which spreads very easily from person to person, mainly through respiratory droplets that infected people cough, sneeze, exhale, sing or talk. It is not regarded as a foodborne disease. From late January 2020 to April 2021, Hong Kong experienced four waves of COVID-19 infections. It was widely reported that many infection clusters were directly or indirectly linked to eating together in close proximity. Given the fact that COVID-19 infection is transmitted through respiratory droplets, it became an urgent task for the Hong Kong government and the public to act to ensure that they were safe in physical and social environments when conducting a variety of activities including social interaction and food consumption. As Hong Kong has the reputation of being a food paradise and the majority of the Hong Kong people consume food outside their home, the public became concerned about the risk of getting infected with COVID-19 as they patronized their favorite food hideouts.

As such, the Hong Kong government has devised strategies to combat the transmission of COVID-19 in the public, while at the same time, the general public has adopted personal strategies to ensure they are safe from COVID-19 infection. At the personal level, some individuals have adjusted their food consumption pattern from one of "eating out" to "eating in".

This chapter examines how individuals in Hong Kong negotiate the correlation between food consumption/food safety and the increase of risk and trust within the framework of food safety studies. In our study, we argue that "trust in people" and "trust in business" play a critical role in enabling Hong Kong people to practice safe eating. At the same time, this chapter also argues that the mobilization and strategic use of thick interpersonal trust and thin trust in business helped to reduce ambiguity and complexity associated with what constitutes a safe shared environment and safe collective group of people for food consumption during the COVID-19 pandemic.

In this chapter, we use a combination of anthropological research methods and a modified form using online media to tap into the views of Hong Kong housewives in their management of fear, risk and trust in relation to food safety

DOI: 10.4324/9781003291220-3

and food consumption within their home environment. We interviewed ten housewives as key informants to hear their views and learn how they utilized trust and distrust in their attempts to reduce risks when eating meals during the COVID-19 pandemic. We held interviews via Zoom meetings to avoid close physical contact and we conducted on-site observations. We also used documentary sources, library research and online information to understand this issue further. The interviewees were chosen using the snowball sampling method. The ten interviews were conducted during the period of November–December 2020. All interviewees were married and lived with their husbands and children in nuclear families, except for one who was single and lived with her widowed mother. These women played the role of "gatekeepers" for home food consumption (McIntosh and Zey 1989). In conducting this research during the COVID-19 pandemic and while Hong Kong society experienced restricted movement and lockdowns, the use of digital technologies and online data collection method has enabled the researchers to continue data collection and understand the difficulties faced by individuals in the local community through empirical studies, albeit in a modified form (Devine et al. 2021, 281).

To understand the real happenings in eating places, on-site observations were conducted on numerous occasions in restaurants, tea houses, Hong Kong-style cafés (*cha chann teng*, 茶餐厅) and other venues from July 2020 to December 2021. This period coincided with the third and fourth waves of outbreak of COVID-19 in Hong Kong that led to preventive measures and problem-solving strategies being implemented and resulted in a change in the behaviors and actions of individuals in these locations. The observations largely concentrated on the activities and interactions of the consumers during the period of dining out. In addition, information about the origin, development and current situation of COVID-19 and local responses in Hong Kong as well as publications on food safety and eating habits in Hong Kong were collected through search online and library research.

Understanding food safety

At the initial outbreak of COVID-19, Chinese media reported a high risk of catching COVID-19 in crowded environments, based on the quick spread of the virus in the city of Wuhan in China – where the first cluster of COVID-19 cases was reported – which was attributed to the hosting of a community banquet of home-made dishes for about 10,000 households (*wanjia* banquet) on January 18, 2020. This event happened five days before the lockdown of Wuhan city (Xu and Liang 2021, 73). Likewise, it was reported that 83 percent of the COVID-19 cluster cases in China were caused by sharing meals among family members (Zuo 2020). However, key public health authorities such as the World Health Organization (WHO), Centers for Disease Control and Prevention (CDC) of USA and food safety assessment authorities such as the European Food Safety Authority (EFSA) and Centre for Food Safety of Hong Kong (CFS) have indicated on their official websites that there is no evidence that food is a COVID-19 transmission route or poses a risk to human health (CDC 2022; CFS 2020; EFSA 2022; WHO 2020). However, in 2020 WHO reminded the public to observe social distancing and avoid crowded eateries and restaurants to prevent COVID-19 transmission in restaurants. This led to heightened public concern and fear in Hong Kong.

In the study of food safety, the focus has been on conditions of food and on naturally harmful or artificial poisonous substances that pose health risks (Kamboj et al. 2020). The food-centered perspective examines food contamination affected by infectious and toxic substances that would be harmful to human health and life when consumed. This is so because "contamination of the food at any stage, from production to consumption, produces bacteria, viruses, parasites, chemical agents and toxins, which eventually cause the foodborne diseases" (Uçar, Yilmaz and Çakıroğlu 2016, 1). With the outbreak of COVID-19, in April 2020, WHO called for effective actions and collaborations of policy makers, food safety regulators, food producers and consumers to ensure food safety to reduce public health risks posed by the foodborne illnesses on its website with special focus on human contact with food in enclosed spaces where it was produced, processed and consumed (WHO 2020).

In recent decades, there has been a growing concern about food hygiene and food safety because of the quick growth of industrial food and the increased eating out practices (Petric 2017; Kamboj et al. 2020; Worsfold 2006). It has been argued that alongside modernity, modern food technologies have led to manufactured risks and hazards/insecurities of commercialized food (Beck 1992; Giddens 1999). Thus, the focus of food safety has long been on food poisoning, food contamination and cross-contamination through food-to-food and person-to-food transmission of bacteria or microbes as well as through eating foods with artificial chemicals and harmful substances (Byrd-Bredbenner et al. 2013; Panghal et al. 2018; Quinlan 2013; Uçar, Yilmaz and Çakıroğlu 2016; Yan 2012; Young et al. 2018). As such, in the area of food studies, the focus has been on the detection of the causes of food contamination/poisoning, reduction of food safety risks, control of foodborne diseases and the implementation of governmental policies and strategies to control risk in food distribution by food handlers and food consumption by consumers respectively.

The treatment of food-related infections and diseases is often regarded as belonging to medical science and public health arena. For example, in 2015, WHO announced that about 31 bacteria, viruses, parasites, toxins and chemicals (including 18 enteric pathogens, ten parasitic diseases and three toxic chemicals) have been identified as factors causing infections in the first report on foodborne diseases (WHO 2015, 125). Studies on foodborne diseases in Hong Kong, Malaysia and mainland China had attributed the cause of these diseases to various factors namely improper food handling that resulted in cross-contamination, poor food hygiene practice by food handlers, food poisoning, lack of public health awareness and eating behavior. This was compounded by the lack of effective state governance, chemical-laden food, widespread use of food additives and pesticides. Finally, climate change and increase in global temperature had led to the rapid growth of pathogens (Chan and Chan 2008; Kamboj et al. 2020; Salleh et al. 2017; Yan 2012).

The increase in processed food and its regular consumption has now become a global norm. As such, global organizations such as WHO, Food and Agriculture Organization of the United Nations and governments have formulated effective laws and policies to handle food-related public health issues and to establish food-related agencies to regulate the food and catering industry (Holley 2010; Kondakci and Zhou 2017; Magnuson et al. 2013). Within the food industry, food operators were "aware of their own role and responsibilities in culture formation and to equip their managers with the skills to create and maintain a positive food safety culture at all levels but particularly at middle management /unit level" (Griffith et al. 2010, 440). At the societal level, there is an increased level of consumer food safety educational interventions and food hygiene training opportunities for food handlers in food industry and consumers to understand food hygiene in food preparation (Evans and Redmond 2014; Milton and Mullan 2010; Byrd-Bredbenner et al. 2013; Young et al. 2018; Insfran-Rivarola et al., 2020).

Management of food safety has become an increasing issue with the rising number of foodborne disease incidences and food poisoning cases caused in part because of new or innovative food technologies and food safety scandals (Almås 1999; Chou and Liou 2010; Rampl et al., 2012; Wilcock et al. 2004; Zagata and Lostak 2012). This has also strongly affected consumers' trust in food and food industry (Sassatelli and Scott 2001; Zachmann and Østby 2011). In recent years in mainland China, incidences related to food safety have affected the trust level of the central, provincial and local governments (Wu, Yang and Chen 2017). Thus, in the food industry, one key concern is to build, rebuild and increase consumer trust (Coveney 2008; Reiher 2017; Yan 2012).

In addition, and especially during the COVID-19 pandemic, food consumption for individuals and the general public has also become an important issue in food safety. Food consumption in public venues, such as restaurants, has now become an important issue in food safety concerns (Salleh et al. 2017, 3). The government and food operators must establish a safe eating environment that the public would trust and patronize. This is significant, as trust has been conceived of as a necessary mechanism for social actors to reduce the complexity of decision-making and allow people to take action (Luhmann [1979] 2017). As such, the conventional food safety studies of contamination and food hygiene have shifted to safe food consumption and safe eating environment that involved not only safe food but also safe social group who eat together. Strict regulatory policies such as controlling the size of the dining groups could help reduce risk of catching infectious diseases during dining (e.g., Coveney 2008; Latvala 2010).

Mobilizing trust and practicing safe eating in Hong Kong amidst COVID-19

In Hong Kong, eating out is a norm and a large majority of the Hong Kong people eat out for breakfast, lunch and dinner in very crowded neighborhood eateries, often known as the Hong Kong's outdoor food stalls (*dai pai dong* 大排档), Hong Kong-style cafés (*cha chann teng*), fast-food joints and restaurants. Today, eating out has become a necessity with fewer families engaged in home cooking. Thus, during the COVID-19 pandemic, this eating out habit has led to the spread of COVID-19 among diners, resulting in a fear and distrust of eating out. If eating out is not possible, buying ready-made food to consume at home is a usual practice. During the pandemic, many Hong Kong people, particularly housewives, have reassessed food consumption options for their family as they are seen as "gatekeepers" of food consumption for the health of the family (McIntosh and Zey 1989).

When a patient had a travel history to Wuhan became the first reported case of COVID-19 in Hong Kong on January 23, 2020, it signaled that the novel coronavirus had begun to spread to Hong Kong. As of December 27, 2021, the Centre for Health Protection (CHP) of Hong Kong declared on its website that the total number of confirmed cases had increased to 12,599. Among these cases, a considerable number of infection clusters were directly or indirectly linked to bars, restaurants, tea houses and even families eating and living under the same roof. For example, the "hotpot gathering cluster" of Kwun Tong District (*The Straits Times*, February 9, 2020), the "bar and band cluster" of the well-known nightlife districts of Lan Kwai Fong, Wan Chai and Tsim Sha Tsui (Adam et al. 2020), the "Bun Kee Noodle and Congee Shop cluster" in Choi Hung (*The Standard*, June 18, 2020), the "Sun Fat Restaurant" in Jordan (*The Standard*, July 10, 2020), the "Kin Wing Canteen cluster" in Tuen Mun (*The Standard*, July 11, 2020), the "Tao Heung at The Pier Market Restaurant cluster" in Mong Kok (*HK01*, August 4, 2020) and many others. It was reported that some chefs and waiters were also infected (*The Standard*, July 11, 2020). It appeared that COVID-19 had infected the food chain and catering industry of Hong Kong (*Time*, May 25, 2020). In this situation, the risk of eating meals in restaurants and even at home increased to a very high level. On the other hand, the information from CFS of Hong Kong and many public health experts showed that it was not necessary to worry about food safety if basic food handling safety measures had been followed, because there was no evidence to suggest that the coronavirus could spread to people through food or food handling (CFS 2020).

As a result, the public had a heightened concern about the risk of eating out and the Hong Kong government rolled out measures on social distancing, shortening the operating hours of restaurants for eating in and the use of "leavehomesafe" app to reduce over-crowdedness in eateries and restaurants (*The Standard*, December 9, 2021). To reduce the risk of COVID-19 infection, working from home and eating in have become "twin measures" to lessen one's fear and risk. Online ordering and food delivery is one way to cope with this pandemic. Likewise, home cooking has also become more popular. Hong Kong housewives, as the home cook and provider of home food, had to engage in food safety practices and negotiate their perceived trust of their food sources in order to ensure safe food consumption at home.

In our studies of housewives as decision-makers in the sourcing and preparation of food, the housewives were involved in negotiating food trust from producers to retailers and consumers in the food environment. As such, there is a three-dimensional analysis of trust (Khodyakov 2007) for the practice of safe food consumption involving "thick" interpersonal trust that concerns the families, close relatives and best friends; "thin" interpersonal trust that concerns people we know and have some information on but do not know well; and institutional trust that deals with businesses. These different levels of trust informed and enabled individuals to make decisions regarding safe eating in various social settings.

Thick interpersonal trust and worry-free eating together

As mentioned earlier, the fast growing of reported cases of COVID-19 related to eating together in Hong Kong made people nervous and worried about contracting novel coronavirus when eating with others in the same place. Because of the strong sense of familism in Chinese culture and society, it was not surprising to find that the high trust among the families might make it possible to practice safe eating at home. As Fukuyama (1995: 88) pointed out, it had long been common for the Chinese not to trust outsiders but to trust only members of their family. All ten interviewees noted that they had made their best efforts to ensure that their families could eat in a healthy and safe environment.

To create a safe environment, all interviewees pointed out that the first and foremost thing was to prevent family members bringing the novel coronavirus back home to reduce the risk of cross-contamination. To achieve this goal, they not only took the necessary preventive measures such as mask-wearing and regular hand cleaning with hand sanitizer, but also asked their family members to change clothes and take a shower immediately when returning home from outside. One interviewee, Mrs. Dong, insisted on taking the strictest precautions to keep the novel coronavirus outside the door of her home to protect her children aged five and one. She explained her experience as follows.

> To avoid person-to-person transmission of the novel coronavirus at home, all the adults in my household, including myself, my husband, my mother-in-law and the domestic helper, must change clothes and take shower at once when coming back from outside. Only after we completely clean our body, we are allowed to take care of the children. For me, even if we just take out the trash in 1 or 2 minutes, we also must take shower and change clothes. I really do this. I know it is time-consuming and not convenient but I believe that it is necessary to avoid contracting the coronavirus. As such, it is very rare for my mother-in-law, our domestic helper and my one-year-old daughter to go downstairs in the past year. It is not easy for them to follow all the precautions.
>
> (Interview on November 23, 2020)

To build trust in others, one can use different strategies to check, to verify and to decide whether to trust or not to trust (Hardin 2001; Heimer 2001). But for family members living and eating together, there is a strong sense of familial obligations, commitments and trust. Under this situation, the potential danger is that when one family member is infected, the others are highly likely to be infected through common residence. Another interviewee, Mrs. Ji, declared that the strong love and high trust of family members enabled them to face and fight against COVID-19 in a collective manner. "If one of our family members gets infected, I am more than happy to accept the fact that all of us will get infected. We love each other very much so we want to face COVID-19 together" (interview on November 21, 2020). As such, the high mutual trust and good hygiene practices helped make the home a safe place in which all the family members could eat with less worry.

Moreover, the "thick" trust among family members facilitated home cooking and eating family meals in the time of COVID-19. All ten interviewees acknowledged that they intentionally minimized the chance of dining out and urged all family members to eat at home. In fact, as the website of EatSmart Restaurant Star+ has shown, eating out was very popular in Hong Kong and people often ate breakfast and lunch in restaurants before the outbreak of COVID-19. After the COVID-19 outbreak, there was a level of distrust among diners sitting in close proximity in restaurants for fear of being infected. As a result, they began to eat more meals at home with families. The interviewees reported that the frequency of home cooking and eating had increased from 50 percent to 80 percent. Apart from the normal practice of cooking dinner at home, the new normal practice was to cook and eat three meals a day at home. Two of the ten interviewees noted that they chose to wake up much earlier in the morning to prepare breakfast so the family members would not take the risk of eating breakfast in the local eateries. They also took the opportunity to cook packed lunch for their family members who worked outside the home to stop them from eating in the crowded eateries. Another interviewee, Mrs. Sun, also believed that it was very important to avoid eating out and do home cooking. During her domestic helper's off-day on Sundays, she would go to the supermarket and buy frozen foods and cook for her family.

When it comes to eating at home, there is a new trend of using serving chopsticks (*gongkuai*, 公筷) and serving food in individual portions (*fencan*, 分餐). It has long been common for the Chinese to share dishes and use personal chopsticks to take food from communal plates. In most cases, sharing food with personal chopsticks is often considered a sociocultural way of strengthening family and social solidarities, as well as a way of fostering high levels of trust among the diners as families, close relatives or best friends. This is to prevent the spread of COVID-19 through saliva droplets. As noted in a *The Wall Street Journal* article on August 11, 2005, medical authorities of Hong Kong had urged the public to use an extra pair of chopsticks as serving chopsticks to minimize the chance of spreading disease since the outbreak of SARS (Severe Acute Respiratory Syndrome) in Hong Kong in 2003. Similar to this, a *South China Morning Post* article on June 14, 2020 noted that the outbreak of COVID-19 made the Chinese government promote the use of serving chopsticks in restaurants. Interviewee Ms. Hou emphasized that she and her mother had developed and maintained the new habit of using serving chopsticks when eating at home from the time of SARS to the current days.

Different from the old cultural notion that viewed serving chopsticks or dividing food into individual servings as too formal, the new understanding expressed by three interviewees revealed that they preferred seeing the new dining practices at home as a way of providing better protection to the loved ones. For example, both Mrs. Ma and Mrs. Dong had followed the strictest precautions to protect the health of their children under the age of ten, so they chose to divide food into small portions and serve individually rather than putting large serving platters on the table to let family members take food with their own chopsticks. For them, this practice was much safer than using serving chopsticks.

Apart from enabling the family members to eat in a relatively safe manner, the "thick" interpersonal trust can also be further extended to explain the willingness of dining together for some close relatives and good friends. Since the COVID-19 pandemic, meeting and eating together with close relatives and good friends was conditioned by the anti-epidemic measures implemented by the government like social distancing measures and size limitations on group gatherings. When the epidemic in Hong Kong eased for a period of time, the social distancing rule and limitations of group gathering were relaxed accordingly. The pre-existing "thick" trust between close relatives and good friends was activated to enable them to have a meal outside their home.

To dine out with friends and relatives, there must be a level of trust during the COVID-19 pandemic. The first type is that of personal trust in the belief that the friends and relatives practice good personal hygiene practice/safe eating habits, while the other type is the system of trust placed on the eating environment (Robbins 2016, 974). The general idea here is that if a close relative or good friend maintained high standards of personal hygiene and took preventive measures, he/she would be regarded as low-risk person and dining with them would pose a low-risk threat of contracting COVID-19. Generally speaking, people were more willing to dine out with a low-risk person. As such, the word "self-disciplined" was mentioned several times when interviewees were asked how to decide with whom to eat during the COVID-19 pandemic. For example, Mrs. Dong stressed the importance of being responsible and self-disciplined.

> To fight against the virus, the most important thing for a single person is to be self-disciplined and try one's best to protect oneself from contracting the coronavirus. Do not affect the others. If everyone makes every effort to protect himself/herself and his/her family very well, the society will not face the severe situation. The real problem is that many people are not responsible for themselves and for the society … I have dined out with very few good friends in the past months. In addition to choosing the high-end restaurant, we also choose those friends who are very self-disciplined. They only take off face mask when eating. They also eat fast. After eating, they put on mask at once. As such, all of us put on mask when we chit-chat. Moreover, I

> require the servers to divide the food into individual servings before putting on the table.
>
> (Interview on November 23, 2020)

It appeared that the new table manner integrated with the key elements of good personal hygiene and safe eating habits had been applied as a standard to decide who could be invited to dine out. Even though individuals had many relatives or friends, only a few of them perceived as having good habits were labeled low-risk and would have the opportunity to eat together. Mrs. Sun shared her experience as follows.

> I am not willing to eat out with friends during this year. For the very few dining together activities, I only dare to eat with the very few best friends with the strong sense of closeness and trustworthiness. One such kind of friend dares to invite me to eat out because she gets to know that I have a habit of preparing lunch box and eating alone in my office. She believes that I am safe. Only when we know each other's living habit very well, we dare to invite the other party to dine out.
>
> (Interview on November 20, 2020)

In this regard, the deep interpersonal trust is reinforced through personal knowledge of the practice of personal hygiene of the family members and friends that led to the individuals considering them as low-risk individuals, fit for socializing purposes that include sharing a meal together in confined spaces. Apart from good living habits of diners, another factor considered is the situational cause; the individuals were compelled to evaluate the importance and urgency of the cause and occasion when being invited to attend a banquet or meal. As interviewee Mrs. Dong indicated:

> It is very popular to get involved into all kinds of social gatherings initiated by colleagues and business partners. I am not willing to join during the epidemic. But if you always refuse to join, it will bring negative impact on your own *guanxi* network. To achieve a balance, now I just choose to take part in one such kind of gathering for socializing purpose in one week.
>
> (Interview on November 23, 2020)

Within the Hong Kong society, individuals tried to achieve a balance between *guanxi* management and health risk management during the COVID-19 pandemic period. As the result of the social distancing policy and the uncertainty and infectiousness of the virus, Hong Kong families and social groups have also restricted the frequency of their socializing and communal dining experiences. Interviewee Ms. Hou noted that the family gatherings of her extended family were reduced to several festive occasions such as the Mid-Autumn Festival and the birthday celebration of her mother during the year, instead of their usual fortnightly gatherings. Likewise, Mrs. Sun also mentioned that she attended only very important event such as a farewell dinner for a friend who was leaving Hong Kong. In other words, the operation of "thick" trust during this pandemic period is compounded by other factors that include risk and food safety in communal gathering and consumption.

To sum up, the thick interpersonal trust provided a foundation for women in Hong Kong to consider when ensuring that communal eating among their social group of selected relatives and friends is safe and risk-free. Thus, selecting those that observed good personal hygiene and practiced social distancing and mask-wearing has become the key criteria in selecting who they would dine with and where they would dine in. It is also dependent on these individuals having a strong sense of mutual responsibility, obligation, support and commitment to ensure that the individuals and the environment are low-risk.

Thin interpersonal trust and protecting against COVID-19 from eating

In contrast to establishing a safe eating environment where individuals eat communally with relatives and close friends that they considered as low-risk, individuals were less likely to have a social meal with non-kin and acquaintances that they considered as high-risk (such as when there was only "thin" interpersonal trust between them). "Thin" interpersonal trust often exists among people we do not know well and are part of the out-group (Khodyakov 2007, 121–123). When Fukuyama compared the trust between family members, kin and non-kin in Chinese societies, he argued that the Chinese usually tended to have strong trust in their families and kin while having low trust in people they do not know well or unrelated people (Fukuyama, 1995, 61–145). In this way, he described Chinese societies as a low-trust society, because the level of spontaneous trusting people of out-groups was relatively low. To elaborate on this point, he provided an example to show that peasants in some villages knew their neighbors, but did not turn to them for help when helping hands were really needed (Fukuyama 1995, 87). Instead, the peasant household chose to be self-dependent and self-sufficient. The possible reason behind this might be that the peasants only had strong trust in people within their own lineage while they had less/low trust in non-lineage village fellows. They usually had no "sense of duties and obligations to anyone outside the family in traditional China" (Fukuyama 1995, 87). As such, in the same Chinese village with multiple lineages, lineage members often have "thin" trust in non-lineage village fellows.

In our Hong Kong case studies, Hong Kong people differentiated between in-group and out-group. Hence, in dealing with the out-group, Hong Kong individuals adopted different coping strategies and protective measures to reduce the chances of being infected with COVID-19. In general, they avoided having meals with those who they did not know well during the pandemic. Among our interviewees, social eating activities had decreased dramatically since the outbreak of COVID-19 especially with people of lower interpersonal trust. For this category, individuals would decline invitations to social meals as there was no strong social obligation to attend. Likewise, they would also stop extending invitations to this out-group. Mrs. Tan stated:

> During the epidemic, it is better for us not to eat together with the others. Before the outbreak of COVID-19, I go to tea house eating with relatives and friends more than ten times one month. This year, I just go one time because of the epidemic. You worry about being infected by the others. Meanwhile, if you make the others catch COVID-19, the government will track down all the people eating together. You get yourself into big trouble.
>
> (Interview on November 17, 2020)

Here, it was the "thin" trust that discouraged people without an intimate relationship from dining together and group gathering in the time of COVID-19. Two interviewees had persuaded their aged mothers to avoid going to tea house for social meals with their elderly friends since the outbreak of COVID-19. While eating breakfast with friends in tea house is a long-established habit of the elderly in Hong Kong, the family members were concerned about the health risks due to the low trust bestowed on the elderly friends of their mother. Another interviewee, Mrs. Lai, pointed out that she had insufficient information about health conditions, personal hygiene and the living environment of her mother's friends, so her trust level in her mother's friends was thin. She explained her concerns as follows.

> Both my mother and mother-in-law love to eat breakfast in tea house. They feel very painful when having no opportunity to do it. So, I accompanied my mum to tea house when the epidemic eased last month. The main reason is that I worry about the health risk when she eats together with others. It is not easy to know clearly who they are, their health condition and the places they have visited. I do not allow my mum to go to tea house with her friends unless the members of family can go with her. I understand she will be very happy to eat breakfast in tea house with her friends. But when they chi-chat loudly, some droplets of saliva may spray into the air and fly here and there. If they really enjoy chatting with others, they may forget to put on mask after eating. As such, I decided to go with her. I will choose the right time slot and the right day, say, around 9 o'clock from Monday to Friday. It is not the peak period because many people have gone to work and the first wave of diners have left. It seems more safe to eat with less people around us. I also explain to my mum why it is safer to go to tea house with family members. The daughters and sons know their own health condition very well and will take preventive measures to protect her. Usually, we put on mask after we eat. Then we can chat with her.
>
> (Interview on November 22, 2020)

It was obvious that the thin trust in her mother's friends forced Mrs. Lai to play an active role in going to tea houses with her mother by herself. The big concern here was the health and hygiene problems of the friends. For Hong Kong people, particularly the elderly, the tea house is not only a place for eating but also a meeting place for families, relatives and friends to exchange information and to chit-chat.

Likewise, the story shared by Ms. Hou showed the risk of eating together with friends in tea house.

> My mum indulges in going to tea house for many decades. When my dad was still alive, he and my mum went to tea house every day, even when No. 8 typhoon signal had been hoisted. It has been a family tradition for my family. It is also very important for the elderly in Hong Kong. So, my mum continues to go to tea house when the number of confirmed cases drops. But she is not so lucky. After she enjoys her breakfast in a tea house in Mong Kok and comes back home, the TV news reports that a confirmed case is a customer of that tea house. My brother, sister and I get to know this piece of news and remind her not to go there again. Although she is not infected, she is scared and stops going to tea house.
>
> (Interview on November 22, 2020)

Facing the real risk of being infected, many people would rethink the necessity of social dining with their relatives or friends. They made decisions based on "thick" and "thin" interpersonal trust levels they have with their social groups. For those inner social groups with thick interpersonal trust, they would likely join in the social dining scene, while for those with thin interpersonal trust, they would likely refrain from joining in. As such, the idea of "thin" interpersonal trust provided a useful framework for people to negotiate their presence in social eating with different groups of people to avoid being exposed to COVID-19 infection.

Comparatively speaking, the trust in business organizations in food and catering industry will probably be much lower than trust in people we do not know well because these businesses are impersonal entities (similar to strangers).

Trust in businesses and safe eating practice

Apart from considering who to dine with, Hong Kong individuals also had to consider the overall environment where food is produced, sold and purchased. Thus, in addition to restaurants and eateries, supermarkets, wet markets and convenience stores there were also places were of high consideration. Hong Kong people would measure these physical spaces in terms of their hygiene conditions and calibrated their trust on these businesses. There are several types of trust in businesses deriving namely that of system trust (Luhmann [1979] 2017), institutional trust (Khodyakov 2007) and consumer trust (Herrera and Blanco 2011; Porral and Levy-Mangin 2016; Rampl et al. 2012). The main idea is that trust in institutions and organizations plays a very important role in facilitating interaction, cooperation and compliance with impersonal institutions. In addition, "institutions can have more resources to provide people with the means of achieving some of their goals" (Khodyakov 2007, 123). Likewise, the food industry at all stages from production onwards has to cultivate consumer trust in order to create a sustainable global food supply chain (Almås 1999; Cook 2001; Herrera and Blanco 2011; Porral and Levy-Mangin 2016; Rampl et al. 2012).

At the consumer level, among those interviewed, safe eating involved dining in restaurants that they considered as trustworthy in terms of cleanliness, hygiene and social distancing of the physical space. At the same time, it also concerns trustworthiness in terms of food preparation by the food handlers and chefs. As such, the middle-class Hong Kong interviewees displayed a higher level of trust in high-end restaurants and the fast-food chains with good reputation. Although the government had urged restaurants to follow social distancing measures, adopt high levels of sanitation, hygiene and food safety regulations, the Hong Kong people often expressed that not all restaurants took the preventive measures seriously and strictly. Among our ten interviewees, three did not believe that the pandemic curbing measures could be fully implemented in restaurants; two of them said that the restaurants could do some but neglected others. Thus, their perceived trust in the restaurants became an important factor for their decision-making in where to eat. Related to this is the perception of the restaurant staff who the interviewees regarded as high risk, given the interaction between them and the diners. Mrs. Ma noted that:

> The servers have to serve many customers during rush hours. Some eaters walk around; some take off mask to eat; some speak. The servers may be contaminated when they serve food to customers or pass platters to eaters. They work in that kind of environment and will transmit the virus to the other eaters.
>
> (Interview on November 22, 2020)

In addition, Mrs. Qiu said food itself was not a big problem but other diners would be a high-risk category capable of transmitting novel coronavirus in restaurants.

> I worry more about customers than food. The big problem is that customers need to take off mask when eating. It is better to eat quickly and put on mask when chatting. Also, when you are eating, many new customers come in. The chance of contacting strangers increases.
>
> (Interview on November 21, 2020)

In this regard, both servers and other diners could be considered as high-risk factors. As such, with social distancing and crowd control in place, many restaurants have spaced their setting arrangements. At the same time, diners also tended to choose restaurants with less customers or avoided eating out during the rush hours. As such, the choice of restaurants in the time of COVID-19 is a reflection of not only one's personal taste, eating habit or preference but also of crowd control and the availability of seats. In addition, these pointed to the level of trust as a critical reference to safe eating places. Here, trust in businesses has led to priority to consume at high-end restaurants and reputable fast-food chain restaurants. For most Hong Kong residents, they perceived high-end restaurants as having the commitment to put in place a well-developed system of food safety and good hygiene practice as well as training and monitoring systems to ensure that the preventive measures would be strictly implemented. It was also believed that the reputable fast-food chain restaurants would have the financial resources to supply anti-epidemic materials to their staff and to increase the frequencies of their cleaning and sanitation of the premise. On the other hand, Hong Kong people viewed some small and medium-sized restaurants as less likely to observe strict hygiene practice strictly as they had less resources and human resources to put in place a full food safety system.

Among our interviewees, four expressed that they would choose high-end restaurants because they felt that this type of restaurant was more trustworthy and safer, with a clean environment with spacious arrangement. Mrs. Ji stressed:

> I like spacious and luxury restaurants because this type of restaurant usually has a professional management team and institutionalized management culture. The top managers can supervise and urge the other staff members to implement the precautions. In contrast, the small restaurants often make every effort to lower the cost so the bosses may neglect some anti-epidemic measures and even want to cut the cost of buying sanitizer. Due to economic recession in the time of COVID-19, some small bosses may lose money and are more likely to go bankrupt. They have no intention to take precautions. On the other side, the big companies have sufficient money to implement preventive measures.
>
> (Interview on November 21, 2020)

Mrs. Dong had the similar viewpoint and emphasized that high-end restaurants could provide hygienic environment and additional services to make eating safer:

> When my best friend and I dine out, we consider the location and targeted customers of the restaurant and precautions taken. We always choose more expensive restaurants, say one thousand Hong Kong dollars per head. So, less people will eat there. This kind of restaurant usually has ample space to leave more space between the tables. We often choose to eat in a private room so the server will divide the food into small portions and serve individually. There is no need for individual person to take food with his own chopstick.
>
> (Interview on November 23, 2020)

As Mrs. Dong has described, more space between tables implied good social distancing practice. Eating in a private room and serving food in individual portions helped reduce the risk of cross-contamination. All these added-value services and potential benefits attracted more high-income people to choose high-end restaurants.

While high-end restaurants cost more, the COVID-19 pandemic has also pushed some lower-middle-income Hong Kongers, who normally do not dine in such places, to consider doing so for the sake of their family safety. Two interviewees, Mrs. Sun and Ms. Hou, acknowledged that they did not dine in luxury restaurants before the outbreak of COVID-19. Ms. Hou rarely ate out but on an occasion when the family did decide to dine out, they were willing to pay a premium for a safe eating environment. Ms. Hou explained her choice as follows.

> When it comes to our big family gathering, we change our habit and choose to eat in luxury Chinese restaurants affiliated with luxury hotels. It is more expensive to eat in this type of restaurant but it is more hygienic. Nowadays, we are more concerned about the cleanliness of the restaurant.
>
> (Interview on November 22, 2020)

For others with a budget to consider, they placed more trust in the local and global fast-food chains than small independent restaurants. The popular fast-food chains mentioned by the informants as trusted restaurants included Maxim's MX, McDonald's, Café de Coral, Fairwood, Saizeriya Italian Restaurant and Tsui Wah Restaurant. Ms. Hou noted that Maxim's MX had maintained at a high level of the hygiene condition and she felt safe buying takeaway food there. Mrs. Ma also buys food from other fast-food restaurants like Saizeriya Italian Restaurant, Fairwood or Tsui Wah Restaurant for her family. Likewise, Mrs. Dong only bought foods from McDonald's.

> McDonald's is a well-known brand so I trust it. McDonald's sells many fried foods. When being fried, the very hot oil helps disinfect the foods. We buy and take the fries away and then eat in an open space.
>
> (Interview on November 23, 2020)

Hong Kong residents based their judgment and trust of the hygiene and food safety conditions of the different restaurants and eateries on their personal consumption experience and on-site observations of the hygiene practice and measures taken by the various restaurants. In this regard, restaurants and eateries need to build trust through avid observation and good practices of hygiene and food safety in order to encourage consumers to enter their doors.

Conclusion

Before COVID-19, the focus on the outbreaks of food scandals, foodborne disease and food poisoning was directed toward the food industry, quality and safety of food as well as the food production environment. To this end, the government has formulated policies and established food safety units to oversee issues of food safety in Hong Kong society. With the onslaught of the COVID-19 pandemic, policies shifted toward the social environment and the food production environment to ensure a safe eating and safe food production environment.

At the same time, given the widespread nature of the infection, interpersonal relationships through group gatherings and group eating have become an important factor to consider. In Hong Kong society, eating out is a part of life and thus safe eating in a safe environment becomes paramount. As such, the Hong Kong people have adopted a careful approach toward their eating habits to ensure safe eating. In this process, understanding the operation of "thick" and "thin" trust in the institution and in the people becomes another key factor to understand how the public measures risk and trust in their practice of safe food and safe eating.

As COVID-19 has ravaged the Hong Kong society and the world for the past two years, different countries have accepted full vaccination as key to eliminating the COVID-19 virus and a policy of coexisting with the virus has emerged. In these countries, society is opening up and functioning as it did pre-COVID-19. Likewise, eateries, bars and public areas are now fully opened in these countries. In Hong Kong, when the government has decided to open up its society, eating and drinking in restaurants, eateries and pubs would again attract crowds of people. But something has changed. The Hong Kong people have now become conscious of food safety and continue to operate safe eating based on a level of interpersonal trust to minimize their personal risk of COVID-19 infection.

Note

1 Khun Eng Kuah is the corresponding author.

References

Adam, Dillon C., Peng Wu, Jessica Y. Wong, Eric H. Y. Lau, Tim K. Tsang, Simon Cauchemez, Gabriel M. Leung, and Benjamin J. Cowling. 2020. "Clustering and Superspreading Potential of SARS-CoV-2 Infections in Hong Kong." *Nature Medicine*, no. 26: 1714–1719. doi: https://doi.org/10.1038/s41591-020-1092-0.

Almås, Reidar. 1999. "Food Trust, Ethics and Safety in Risk Society." *Sociological Research Online* 4(3): 275–281. doi: https://doi.org/10.5153/sro.337.

Beck, Ulrich. 1992. *Risk Society: Towards a New Modernity*. London: Sage Publications.

Byrd-Bredbenner, Carol, Jacqueline Berning, Jennifer Martin-Biggers, and Virginia Quick. 2013. "Food Safety in Home Kitchens: A Synthesis of the Literature." *International Journal of Environmental Research and Public Health* 10(9): 4060–4085. doi: https://doi.org/10.3390/ijerph10094060.

Chan, S.F. and Z.C.Y. Chan. 2008. "A *Review* of *Foodborne Disease Outbreaks* From *1996* to *2005* In *Hong Kong* and *Its Implications* on *Food Safety Promotion*", *Journal of Food Safety 28*(2): 276–299. doi: https://doi.org/10.1111/j.1745-4565.2008.00120.x.

Chou, Kuei-tien, and Hwa-meei Liou. 2010. "'System Destroys Trust?': Regulatory Institutions and Public Perceptions of Food Risks in Taiwan." *Social Indicators Research* 96(1): 41–57. doi: https://doi.org/10.1007/s11205-009-9465-2

CDC (Centers for Disease Control and Preventions of USA). 2022. *Food safety and Coronavirus Disease 2019 (COVID-19)*. https://www.cdc.gov/foodsafety/newsletter/food-safety-and-Coronavirus.html

CFS (Centre for Food Safety of Hong Kong). 2020. *Food safety advice on prevention of COVID-19 and FAQs*. https://www.cfs.gov.hk/english/whatsnew/files/Food_Safety_Advice_on_Prevention_of_COVID-19_and_FAQs_rev_20200228.pdf

Cook, Karen S. 2001. "Trust in society." In *Trust in Society*, edited by Karen S. Cook, xi–xxvii. New York: Russell Sage Foundation.

Coveney, John. 2008. "Food and Trust in Australia: Building a Picture." Public Health Nutrition 11(3): 237–245. doi: https://doi.org/10.1017/S1368980007000250.

Devine, Daniel, Jennifer Gaskell, Will Jennings, and Gerry Stoker. 2021. "Trust and the Coronavirus Pandemic: What are the Consequences of and for Trust? An Early Review of the Literature.", *Political Studies Review* 19(2): 274–285. doi: https://doi.org/10.1177/1478929920948684.

EFSA (European Food Safety Authority). 2022. *EFSA and COVID-19*. https://www.efsa.europa.eu/en/topics/efsa-and-covid-19

Evans, Ellen W., and Elizabeth C. Redmond. 2014. "Behavioral Risk Factors Associated with Listeriosis in the Home: A Review of Consumer Food Safety Studies." *Journal of Food Protection* 77(3): 510–521. doi: https://doi.org/10.4315/0362-028X.JFP-13-238.

Fukuyama, Francis. 1995. *Trust: The Social Virtues and the Creation of Prosperity*. London: Hamish Hamilton.

Giddens, Anthony. 1999. "Risk and Responsibility." *Modern Law Review* 62(1): 1–10. doi: https://doi.org/10.1111/1468-2230.00188.

Griffith, C.J., K.M. Livesey, and D. Clayton. 2010. "The Assessment of Food Safety Culture." *British Food Journal* 112(4): 439–456. doi: https://doi.org/10.1108/00070701011034448.

Hardin, Russell. 2001. "Conceptions and Explanations of Trust." In *Trust in Society*, edited by Karen S. Cook, 3–39. New York: Russell Sage Foundation.

Heimer, Carol A. 2001. "Solving the Problem of Trust." In *Trust in Society*, edited by Karen S. Cook, 40–88. New York: Russell Sage Foundation.

Herrera, Carmina Fandos, and Carlos Flavián Blanco. 2011. "Consequences of Consumer Trust in PDO Food Products: The Role of Familiarity." *Journal of Product & Brand Management* 20(4): 282–296. doi: https://doi.org/10.1108/10610421111148306.

Holley, Richard A. 2010. "Smarter Inspection will Improve Food Safety in Canada." *Canadian Medical Association Journal* 182(5): 471–473. doi: https://doi.org/10.1503/cmaj.090517.

Insfran-Rivarola, Andrea, Diego Tlapa, Jorge Limon-Romero, Yolanda Baez-Lopez, Marco Miranda-Ackerman, Karina Arredondo-Soto, and Sinue Ontiveros. 2020. "A Systematic Review and Meta-Analysis of the Effects of Food Safety and Hygiene Training on Food Handlers." *Foods* 9(9): 1–24. doi: https://doi.org/10.3390/foods9091169.

Kamboj, Sahil, Neeraj Gupta, Julie D. Bandral, Garima Gandotra and Nadira Anjum. 2020. "Food Safety and Hygiene: A Review." *International Journal of Chemical Studies* 8(2): 358–368. doi: 10.22271/chemi.2020.v8.i2f.8794.

Khodyakov, Dmitry. 2007. "Trust as a Process: A Three-Dimensional Approach." *Sociology* 4(1): 115–132. doi: https://doi.org/10.1177/0038038507072285.

Kondakci, Turkay and Weibiao Zhou. 2017. "Recent Applications of Advanced Control Techniques in Food Industry." *Food and Bioprocess Technology* 10(3): 522–542. doi: https://doi.org/10.1007/s11947-016-1831-x.

Latvala, Terhi. 2010. "Risk, Information, and Trust in the Food Chain: Factors Explaining Consumer Willingness to Pay." *International Journal on Food System Dynamics* 4: 295–304.

Luhmann, Niklas. (1979) 2017. *Trust and Power*. Reprint, Cambridge: Polity Press.

Magnuson, Bernadene, Ian Munro, Peter Abbot, Nigel Baldwin, Rebecca Lopez-Garcia, Karen Ly, Larry McGirr, Ashley Roberts, and Susan Socolovsky. 2013. "Review of The Regulation and Safety Assessment of Food Substances in Various Countries and Jurisdictions." *Food Additives & Contaminants: Part A* 30(7): 1147–1220. doi: https://doi.org/10.1080/19440049.2013.795293.

McIntosh, Wm. Alex, and Mary Zey. 1989. "Women as Gatekeepers of Food Consumption: A Sociological Critique." *Food and Foodways* 3(4): 317–332.

Milton, Alyssa, and Barbara Mullan. 2010. "Consumer Food Safety Education for The Domestic Environment: A Systematic Review." *British Food Journal* 112(9): 1003–1022. doi: https://doi.org/10.1108/00070701011074363.

Panghal, Anil, Navnidhi Chhikara, Neelesh Sindhu, and Sundeep Jaglan. 2018. "Role of Food Safety Management Systems in Safe Food Production: A review." *Journal of Food Safety* 38(4): 1–11. doi: https://doi.org/10.1111/jfs.12464.

Petrick, Gabriella. 2017. "Industrial Food." In *The Oxford Handbook of Food History*, edited by Jeffrey M. Pilcher, 258–278. New York: Oxford University Press.

Porral, Cristina Calvo and Levy-Mangin, Jean-Pierre 2016 "Food Private Label Brands: The Role of Consumer Trust on Loyalty and Purchase Intention." *British Food Journal* 118(3): 679–696. doi: https://doi.org/10.1108/BFJ-08-2015-0299.

Quinlan, Jennifer J. 2013. "Foodborne Illness Incidence Rates and Food Safety Risks for Populations of Low Socioeconomic Status and Minority Race/Ethnicity: A Review of the Literature." *International Journal of Environmental Research and Public Health* 10(8): 3634–3652. doi: 10.3390/ijerph10083634.

Rampl, Linn Viktoria, Tim Eberhardt, Reinhard Schütte, and Peter Kenning. 2012. "Consumer Trust in Food Retailers: Conceptual Framework and Empirical Evidence." *International Journal of Retail & Distribution Management* 40(4): 254–272. doi: https://doi.org/10.1108/09590551211211765.

Reiher, Cornelia. 2017. "Food Safety and Consumer Trust in Post-Fukushima Japan." *Japan Forum* 29(1): 53–76. doi: https://doi.org/10.1080/09555803.2016.1227351.

Robbins, Blaine G. 2016. "What is Trust? A Multidisciplinary Review, Critique, and Synthesis." *Sociology Compass* 10(10): 972–986. doi: https://doi.org/10.1111/soc4.12391.

Salleh, Wahida, Mohd Nizam Lani, Wan Zawiah Wan Abdullah, Tuan Zainazor Tuan Chilek, and Zaiton Hassan. 2017. "A Review on Incidences of Foodborne Diseases and Interventions for A Better National Food Safety System in Malaysia." *Malaysian Applied Biology* 46(3): 1–7.

Sassatelli, Roberta. and Alan Scott. 2001. "Novel Food, New Markets and Trust Regimes: Responses to the Erosion of Consumers' Confidence in Austria, Italy and the UK." *European Societies* 3(2): 213–244. doi: https://doi.org/10.1080/14616690120054339.

Uçar, Aslı, Mustafa Volkan Yilmaz, and Funda Pınar Çakıroğlu. 2016. "Food Safety-Problems and Solutions." In *Significance, Prevention and Control of Food Related Diseases*, edited by Hussaini Anthony Makun, 1–25. London: IntechOpen.

Wilcock, Anne, Maria Pun, Joseph Khanona, and May Aung. 2004. "Consumer Attitudes, Knowledge and Behaviour: A Review of Food Safety Issues." *Trends in Food Science & Technology* 15(2): 56–66. doi: https://doi.org/10.1016/j.tifs.2003.08.004.

WHO (World Health Organization). 2015. *WHO Estimates of the Global Burden of Foodborne Diseases: Foodborne Disease Burden Epidemiology Reference Group 2007–2015*. https://apps.who.int/iris/handle/10665/199350.

WHO (World Health Organization). 2020. *Food Safety*. https://www.who.int/en/news-room/fact-sheets/detail/food-safety.

Worsfold, Denise. 2006. "Eating Out: Consumer Perceptions of Food Safety." *International Journal of Environmental Health Research* 16(3): 219–229. doi: https://doi.org/10.1080/09603120600641417.

Wu, Xiaolong, Dali L. Yang, and Lijun Chen. 2017. "The Politics of Quality-of-Life Issues: Food Safety and Political Trust in China." *Journal of Contemporary China* 26(106): 601–615. doi: https://doi.org/10.1080/10670564.2017.1274827.

Xu, Lanlan, and Yuqing Liang. 2021. "COVID-19 in Mainland China: Anti-epidemic Social Mobilization Under Comprehensive Management." In *Facts and Analysis: Canvassing COVID-19 Responses*, edited by Linda Chelan Li, 71–88. Hong Kong: City University of Hong Kong Press.

Yan, Yunxiang. 2012. "Food Safety and Social Risk in Contemporary China." *The Journal of Asian Studies* 71(3): 705–729. doi: https://doi.org/10.1017/S0021911812000678.

Young, Ian, Abhinand Thaivalappil, Judy Greig, Richard Meldrum, and Lisa Waddell. 2018. "Explaining the Food Safety Behaviours of Food Handlers Using Theories of Behaviour Change: A Systematic Review." *International Journal of Environmental Health Research* 28(3): 323–340. doi: https://doi.org/10.1080/09603123.2018.1476846.

Zachmann, Karin, and Per Østby. 2011. "Food, Technology, and Trust: An Introduction." *History and Technology* 27(1): 1–10. doi: https://doi.org/10.1080/07341512.2011.548970.

Zagata, Lukas, and Michal Lostak. 2012. "In Goodness We Trust. The Role of Trust and Institutions Underpinning Trust in the Organic Food Market." *Sociologia Ruralis* 52(4): 470–487. doi: https://doi.org/10.1111/j.1467-9523.2012.00574.x.

Zou, Mandy. 2020. "As Covid-19 changes chopstick habits, China's diners ponder how to keep family love and intimacy alive" *South China Morning Post*, June 14. https://www.scmp.com/news/china/society/article/3088830/covid-19-changes-chopstick-habits-diners-ponder-how-keep-family

4 State-led COVID-19 governance and the negotiation of trust in local Chinese communities in the Greater Bay Area of China

Khun Eng Kuah[1] and Hong Jin

Introduction

In November 2019, a new coronavirus, commonly called COVID-19, first emerged in Wuhan and spread rapidly to the rest of China, leading to the first lockdown of the city of Wuhan. The COVID-19 pandemic was seen as a public health risk and created mayhem, stress and uncertainty, leading to public distrust of the inability of the government and the public health sector to handle this pandemic.

To combat the public health risk brought about by this pandemic, mainland Chinese governments developed a COVID-19 governance framework with directives from the central government authority and its team of medical experts while the actual implementation was assigned and managed by the provincial, municipal and local governments. This top-down approach with strict instruction to eliminate the COVID-19 virus at all costs and attain a zero infection rate had led to the swift containment of the COVID-19 infection in China.

At the same time, the Chinese government has also embarked on a massive public relations campaign to convince its citizens and the wider world of its efforts in containing the COVID-19 pandemic and to rebuild trust in the government. Things turned a corner following the success of containing the spread of COVID-19 in China, with the public reassessing their trust and value of the government-led COVID-19 strategies and actions.

This chapter examines the implementation of COVID-19 policy and governance and the related issues of fear, risk and trust of local residents and communities in the Shenzhen and Guangzhou districts of the Greater Bay Area of China as they faced the COVID-19 pandemic. It explores how the residents of the local community negotiated and constructed compliance with the state-directed strategies and actions. It also explores how the public shifted their attitude from the initial trust deficit to one of trust surplus toward the Chinese authorities and leaders in the management and containment of the COVID-19 pandemic.

This chapter relied on numerous documentary sources, media reports as well as formal ethnographic interviews of 11 informants and participant observations of two local communities in the city of Shenzhen and a local community in Guangzhou in the Greater Bay Area of China as well as personal experiences. As the COVID-19 pandemic was still ongoing at the time of writing this chapter, both

DOI: 10.4324/9781003291220-4

authors have experienced lockdown and compulsory mass nucleic acid testing in their local community, in addition to numerous rounds of health status checks as they traveled out of their local community to other communities in the same city or across the city and faced compulsory quarantine upon returning from abroad.

Negotiating fear and trust with the multi-level COVID-19 governance framework

When the COVID-19 pandemic first broke out in the city of Wuhan, it was traced to the Wuhan Huanan Sea Food Wholesale Market (武汉华南海鲜批发市场) where seafood and wildlife animals were sold. In the beginning, it was accepted that this was where the pandemic broke out. As COVID-19 infections spread globally, many conspiracy theories pointed to human errors, rather than the scientific ones that claimed coronavirus originated in wildlife.[2] Since then, with the global explosion of the COVID-19 and the development of the new strains, much attention has been focused on containing it through vaccination. With a large proportion of the population vaccinated, many parts of the world have started to adopt the strategy of coexisting with the COVID-19 virus and treating it as an endemic rather than a pandemic. Mainland China, on the other hand, continued to uphold the zero-infection and shifting it in mid-2022 to dynamic zero-infection strategy.

During the initial months after the Wuhan outbreak, China was not prepared for the scale and rapid transmission of the COVID-19 infection that led to a countrywide lockdown in early 2020. During this period, there was much confusion and a generally lacking, poor response. As such, there was widespread dissatisfaction and suspicion of government strategies and actions and doubt about the ability of the government to control COVID-19 infections. This had led to a high level of distrust of the government and the information released at the central, provincial and local levels.

To better manage and contain COVID-19, the central government devised and activated a three-tier national public health system to battle against the spread of the virus. This system was first established after the SARS outbreak in 2013 and it is a multi-level system of public health governance that involved government bureaucracies and public health institutions at central, provincial, municipal and local levels.

Within the mainland Chinese authoritarian political system, all decisions were top-driven while the actual acts on the ground were devolved to regional and local level governments (Liu et al. 2021). In this COVID-19 pandemic environment, China's emergency public health system and COVID-19 governance reflected a tightly centralized control with policies and actions directed from the top while the implementations of the policy delegated to the provincial and lower levels of government. As such, failure to eliminate or control the spread of the virus became the responsibility of the local governments as China continued its COVID-19 zero-infection policy. At the end of 2021, after a hiatus of zero infection, COVID-19 cases were detected among the residents of the local community in the city of Xian that spread to neighboring provinces, and two senior

Communist officials were removed because of their inability to bring the infection under control (*Straits Time*, January 3, 2022, "Coronavirus: China removes two officials from Xian", https://www.straitstimes.com/asia/east-asia/coronavirus-china-removes-two-officials-from-xian, accessed January 23, 22). The multi-level COVID-19 governance framework involved governments at different levels. At the top level, different ministries under the State Council were involved in policymaking, devising strategies and coordinating decisions on the types of actions required. One key decision-making body is the National Health Commission of the People's Republic of China (NHC), and together with its sub-division of the Disease Prevention and Control Bureau, was responsible for devising strategies and policies as well as preventive plans and measures to stop the infection. It was also responsible for decisions about COVID-19 data releases and regulating all public hospitals in relation to COVID-19 patients and quarantine rules. The Ministry of Industry and Information Technology was responsible for the control and dissemination of the big data and mobile technology and put in place the trace and track system. Through the use of the mobile phone geolocation app via the Beidou satellite system, the government was able to collect travel information and movements of individuals to rapidly track and trace and quarantine COVID-19 infected individuals. It also used the ubiquitous social media outlet WeChat as a communicative channel to inform the general public of the infected districts and isolate these districts with rapid speed. At the same time, the government ministries also used data from public health sectors, customs, immigration control bureaus and public transportation centers (such as civil aviation and railways) to generate enormous digital footprints on the movements of its population. These data were fed into the National Government Service Platform with real name authentication that enabled authorities to obtain instant records of an individual's travel record from the past 14 days, vaccination status and the results of nucleic acid tests. The data were also placed on the individual's digital travel card and digital health card and made accessible through the apps on their mobile phone. Individuals were required to log onto their digital travel and health cards to show their COVID-19 status whenever they boarded a train, entered hospitals, shopping malls, restaurants or any public areas. The Ministry of Industry and Information Technology also advocated the use of artificial intelligence and 5G technology for remote diagnosis and treatment, as well as using thermographic scanning at railway stations and airports to detect signs of fever among crowds, a practice in line with the global trend.

The extensive deployment of technological surveillance and control has contributed to the rapid control of the COVID-19 transmission. Like elsewhere in the world, it also raised the issue of data control and individual privacy breach. However, in China, the authoritarian system did not allow for public criticism and resistance. Liu and Zhao (2021) attributed it to the prevalent guardianship discourse in China that gave rulers certain discretionary power, the sociocultural imagination where technology was closely associated with nation building and rejuvenation, as well as a compliance tradition that explained people's tolerance of such surveillance. At the same time, the authoritarian regime did not tolerate dissent and critics were punished for speaking out. Hence, among the population, the fear of being subjected to punishment for public criticism and resistance has led to a docile population that followed obediently.

On a second level, the implementation of COVID-19 strategies was delegated to provincial, municipal and local governments that have responsibility for different levels of powers to carry out the duties of eliminating COVID-19. Provincial and municipal governments decided on the implementation of concrete measures and strategies such as the quarantine rules, management of community and population movements, all in accordance with the central guidelines. It was also their responsibility to transmit the COVID-19 strategies to local leaders in neighborhood communities and to monitor the process and implementation of the policies within their jurisdiction.

The multi-level governance system enabled coordination and implementation of policy and strategies of different government agencies and private sectors across tiers, territories and sectors (Liu et al. 2021). This coordinated effort across the spectrum would enable the quick containment of the spread of COVID-19 and the attainment of zero infection. In addition, it also acted as a discursive force of governmentality that disseminated information and shaped people's knowledge of COVID-19, influenced their perception of risk and their negotiation process of trust and distrust of the government.

Community governance and policy implementation

On a third level, urban community administrative divisions consist of the Community Communist Party, sub-district offices and workstations. At this level, it is the Community Communist Party that holds overall responsibility and ultimate authority over community issues. Under it is the sub-district office where its role is management control while the workstation coordinates the actual policy implementation. At each urban community level, the workstation – together with the police office and the healthcare center – constituted the "three-in-one" local management system and acted as the "local agencies of the state", representing the penetrative power of the central government into the grassroots neighborhoods (Zhu et al. 2021). These local agencies of the state have played a leading role in enforcing governance and mobilizing local organizations such as business corporations, property management companies and NGOs to ensure that COVID-19 strategies were implemented, and the public complied with them in a timely and rigorous manner.

At the urban community level, the local community was divided according to a grid governance system.[3] Local community is also commonly known as a neighborhood that comprised residential complexes, schools, health centers and stores where people live their daily lives. It is also a jurisdiction management unit in China's grid governance system.

This system was first established in 2013 after it was advocated in the Third Plenary Session of the 18th CPC Central Committee as a management system to improve the social management of local institutions and grassroots communities

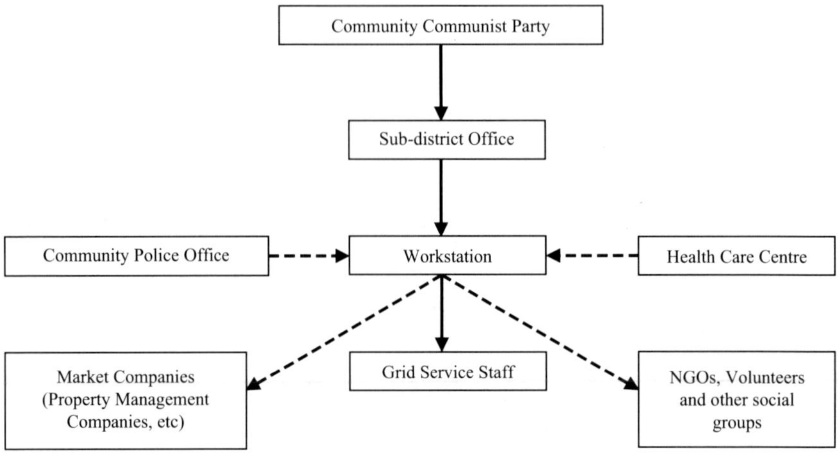

Figure 4.1 The Structure of Government Agencies and Social Organizations at Local Community Level Note: The direction of solid black lines indicates administrative affiliation. The dotted black lines indicate coordination and cooperation. Sub-district Office is called *jie dao ban* (街道办) in Chinese; workstation refers to *shequ gongzuozhan* (社区工作站) in Chinese; and grid service staff is called *wangge gongzuo renyuan* (网格工作人员) in Chinese.

in urban cities. The grid governance system referred to an administrative division of urban neighborhoods into smaller units to enable active and timely management and intervention through routine inspection and surveillance. Before the COVID-19 pandemic, local governments have already recruited a large number of grassroots workers to carry out work on the ground based on the individual grid. This enabled the workers to reach quickly to the individuals in the local communities during the pandemic (see Figure 4.1).

Under the grid governance system, the management and governance of COVID-19 control reached down to almost all the work units or *danwei* community, street residential community and commercial residential community (Li 2020).[4] In our case study of an affluent gated commercial residential community, a working-class street residential community in Shenzhen and a gated middle-class residential community in Guangzhou, strict control and detailed regulations were implemented at the local community level that regulated the behavior, actions and movements of the residents in these three communities. These strict control and regulatory requirements also impacted the perception of the risk of COVID-19 among the local population.

Xin is a working-class street residential community/neighborhood governed by the Xin workstation. It covered a mixed industrial and residential area in a Shenzhen suburb. It has around 700 permanent residents and more than 30,000 low-income rural migrant workers. According to a workstation officer in Xin community, during the COVID-19 outbreak in early 2020, all workstation staff had to follow a strict working protocol with policy directives transmitted from the Shenzhen municipal government. For example, they were required to form inspection teams to conduct patrols and thorough inspections in the Xin community. Each team comprised four members: one doctor from a healthcare center, one police officer, one workstation officer and one grid worker. Each was assigned with a clear responsibility: doctors were tasked with body temperature checks; police officers were responsible for maintaining order; workstation officers were to collect travel information and social contacts of the residents. The buildings in this neighborhood were mostly constructed by the villagers for the rural migrant workers who lived and work there. This was the phenomenon of "village in the urban setting" (*chengzhongcun*城中村) where the neighborhood was organically built through the years and hence appeared disorganized and chaotic. It was incorporated into the grid governing system. Under this system, grid members on the ground had mastered detailed information of the households and migrant workers. During the COVID-19 outbreak, the grid members were able to guide members of the work teams to each household for inspection. They were also able to help control the movement of the residents in and out of the community by directing them through one entrance and closing the other entry points. In contrast, the gated upper middle-class commercial and residential Yan community engaged a property management company to enforce gate control, conduct information check and exit and entry of its residents. Likewise, the Jida neighborhood community had also security guards checking on the exit and entry of the residents to ensure that outsiders were prevented from entering the neighborhood. When it was detected that there were a couple of infected cases, the local authorities organized mass nucleic acid tests for all members including young children. Also, when there were infected cases detected in other cities, the Guangzhou city government's instruction was for all non-essential travel outside the province.

According to the workstation officer in Xin community, the property service company manager in Yan community and the security guard at the Jida community, these COVID-19 regulations were meticulous and detailed including temperature check, gate control, daily disinfection, in-field key group inspection, information collection and quarantine management. In response to the changing situation of virus transmission, preventive measures were adjusted frequently at the municipal level and then transmitted to workstation staff and company managers through meetings, phone calls and paperwork.

Grassroots officers faced enormous pressure in implementing the COVID-19 policy as the state government held them responsible for any failure and ineffective control.[5] During the outbreak, they had to follow a harsh regime and a strict timeline to complete the required tasks. According to the workstation officer, during the outbreak, if there were residents returning from high-risk zones (those regions that have infected COVID-19 cases) or failed to provide detailed travel information, workstation members were required to reach these residents within 30 minutes after they entered into the community. According to him, "such cases had to be inspected immediately, without any delay and even during midnight".

The tight control and multi-level COVID-19 governance left little space for autonomy for local communities to take initiatives, but there was shared responsibility between the community government agencies and the commercial sector where in the case of the Xin community, the workstation outsourced the task of disinfection to a market company and contacted factories and companies for supply of masks. "The integrative connections between government and market sectors demonstrate an administrative mechanism featuring the sharing of social resources" (Zhu et al. 2021, 13).

Before the pandemic, commercial housing as a gated neighborhood enjoyed certain autonomy from government surveillance due to a controlled gate, exclusive use of enclosed space and the presence of a property service company that served the residents in the community. However, this arrangement was broken as a result of the pandemic (Zhu et al. 2021). According to a property manager, the property company could no longer perform its tasks autonomously but had to comply with government preventive measures. Further, he stated that

> the workstation required us to disinfect public space daily but did not give any more details. We set up a protocol of disinfecting every two hours during the most critical time. It also required us to handle rubbish from quarantined families separately. We wrapped their rubbish with plastic bags and put in a rubbish bin labeled from quarantined families. In addition, at the very beginning, the workstation did not distribute any banners or posters for raising awareness on COVID-19 and its preventive measures, and we took initiative to design and hang up such banners with slogan such as 'before, only bad persons wear a mask; now, good neighbors wear a mask'. We also persuaded residents to return home when they walked out without wearing a mask. This was not required by the government at that time, but we put it into practice. In some way, we worked ahead of governments in COVID-19 management.

As this case illustrates, there was still room for individual initiatives as long as they fell within the framework of the COVID-19 governance laid out by the government. In this way, the property management followed the instructions provided and took on the responsibility of policing the residents to ensure COVID-19 compliance, thus it was seen as proactively supporting government policies and not contradicting them (see Figures 4.2 and 4.3).

Explicit instructions on COVID-19 prevention were provided for the working-class Xin community. Besides posters and banners hanging at the entrance and inside the buildings, a loudspeaker was installed in the street that repeatedly broadcast preventive measures to extoll the residents to maintain social distancing and observe personal hygiene such as handwashing. The use of propaganda tools is not new. It has been a common tactic used by the CCP to educate the population and regulate their behaviors through continuous broadcasting of desirable policies and ideologies at the local community level and, increasingly, through social media. During the COVID-19 pandemic, this well-established broadcasting tool was used widely in local communities. This practice continued even as the

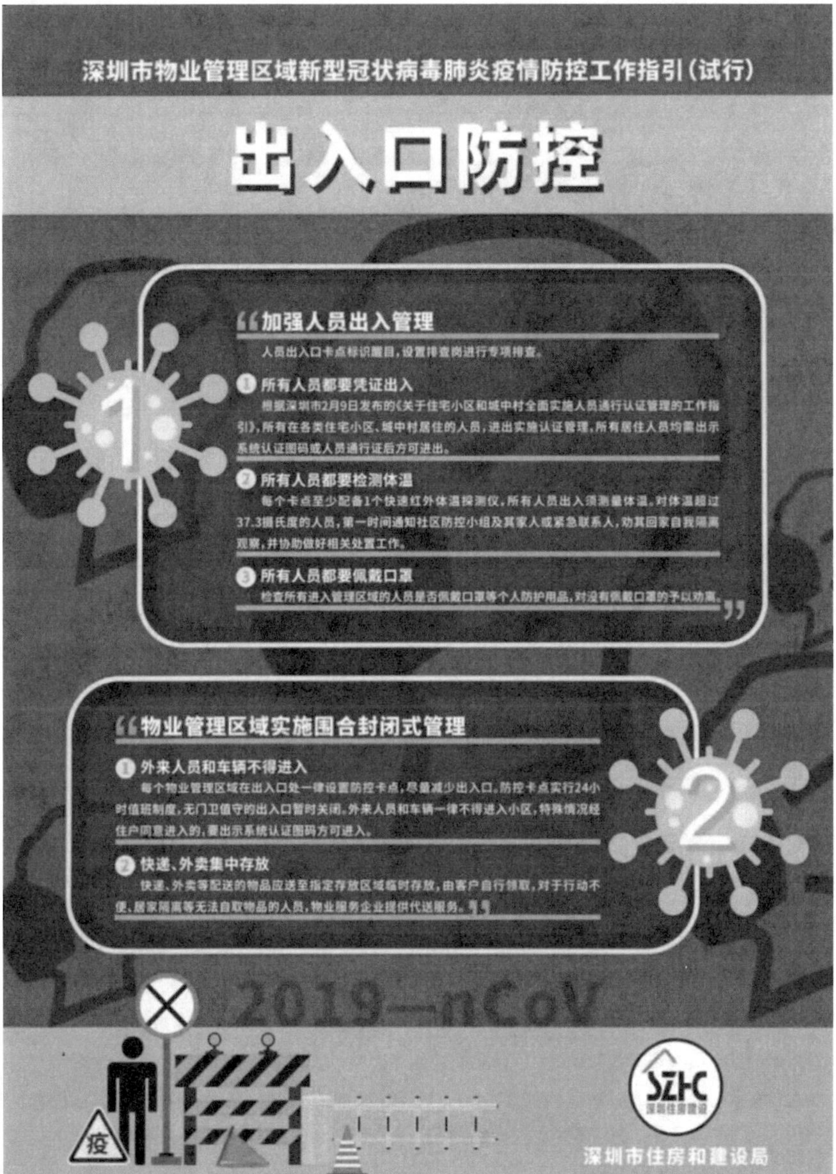
深圳市物业管理区域新型冠状病毒肺炎疫情防控工作指引（试行）
出入口防控
加强人员出入管理
人员出入口卡点标识醒目，设置排查岗进行专项排查。
1 所有人员都要凭证出入
根据深圳市2月9日发布的《关于住宅小区和城中村全面实施人员通行认证管理的工作指引》，所有在各类住宅小区、城中村居住的人员，进出实施认证管理，所有居住人员均需出示系统认证图码或人员通行证后方可进出。
2 所有人员都要检测体温
每个卡点至少配备1个快速红外体温探测仪，所有人员出入须测量体温。对体温超过37.3摄氏度的人员，第一时间通知社区防控小组及其家人或紧急联系人，劝其回家自我隔离观察，并协助做好相关处置工作。
3 所有人员都要佩戴口罩
检查所有进入管理区域的人员是否佩戴口罩等个人防护用品，对没有佩戴口罩的予以劝离。
物业管理区域实施围合封闭式管理
1 外来人员和车辆不得进入
每个物业管理区域在出入口处一律设置防控卡点，尽量减少出入口。防控卡点实行24小时值班制度，无门卫值守的出入口暂时关闭。外来人员和车辆一律不得进入小区，特殊情况经住户同意进入的，要出示系统认证图码方可进入。
2 快递、外卖集中存放
快递、外卖等配送的物品应送至指定存放区域临时存放，由客户自行领取，对于行动不便、居家隔离等无法自取物品的人员，物业服务企业提供代送服务。
2019-nCoV
疫
SZHC
深圳市住房和建设局

Figure 4.2 A poster directing entry/exit in Yan community. Photo taken by Hong Jin.

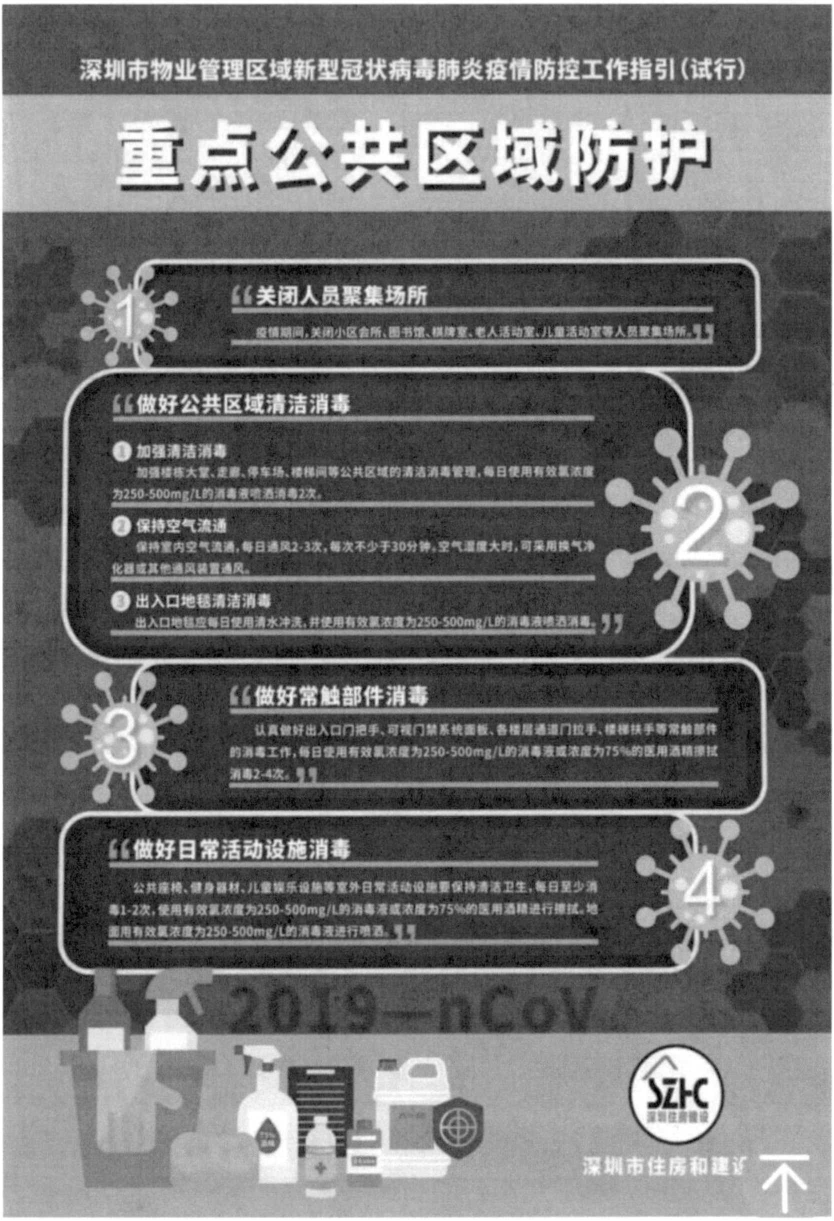
深圳市物业管理区域新型冠状病毒肺炎疫情防控工作指引（试行）
重点公共区域防护
1
关闭人员聚集场所
疫情期间，关闭小区会所、图书馆、棋牌室、老人活动室、儿童活动室等人员聚集场所。
2
做好公共区域清洁消毒
加强清洁消毒
加强楼栋大堂、走廊、停车场、楼梯间等公共区域的清洁消毒管理，每日使用有效氯浓度为250-500mg/L的消毒液喷洒消毒2次。
保持空气流通
保持室内空气流通，每日通风2-3次，每次不少于30分钟。空气湿度大时，可采用换气净化器或其他通风装置通风。
出入口地毯清洁消毒
出入口地毯应每日使用清水冲洗，并使用有效氯浓度为250-500mg/L的消毒液喷洒消毒。
3
做好常触部件消毒
认真做好出入口门把手、可视门禁系统面板、各楼层通道门拉手、楼梯扶手等常触部件的消毒工作，每日使用有效氯浓度为250-500mg/L的消毒液或浓度为75%的医用酒精擦拭消毒2-4次。
4
做好日常活动设施消毒
公共座椅、健身器材、儿童娱乐设施等室外日常活动设施要保持清洁卫生，每日至少消毒1-2次，使用有效氯浓度为250-500mg/L的消毒液或浓度为75%的医用酒精进行擦拭。地面用有效氯浓度为250-500mg/L的消毒液进行喷洒。
2019—nCoV
SZHC
深圳市住房和建设

Figure 4.3 A poster on key policies on COVID-19 control hanging in Yan community. Photo taken by Hong Jin.

COVID-19 virus had largely subsided in Shenzhen. This tactic, however, was not used in the tranquil middle-class Yan neighborhood. This difference in treatment betrayed a prejudice against migrant workers where they were usually perceived as less educated and hence less informed, vigilant and knowledgeable. Thus, they needed to be reminded continuously of the expected policies and their personal hygiene and practices.

Two years after the outbreak of the COVID-19 pandemic, China's aggressive and intensive preventive measures had been successful for a variety of reasons. The grid governance system enabled rapid deployment of numerous agents on the ground to implement the policies and take required actions. This, coupled with the presence and strong control of local government agencies at the community level, has led to a prolonged period of zero infection rate country-wide until the end of 2021 where COVID-19 infectious clusters again emerged throughout China.

Fear, risk and distrust during the COVID-19 outbreak

The global COVID-19 pandemic, its infectious nature, rapid transmissibility and mortality rates have led to fear and heightened the level of distrust by the individuals and the local community toward the government and health agencies over the risk of being infected by the virus. From the structure and system perspective, risk in modernity does not derive from consequences of natural hazards; rather, it is embedded in the modernization process, produced by society's preoccupation with the future (Beck 1992; Giddens 1998). Another school of thought gives attention to the social–cultural impact on people's perception of risk, conceptualizing it as a result of construction and negotiation with society and cultural worldviews (Douglas 1992). A novel and contagious virus such as COVID-19 poses a risk to both people's health and their social life, yet perception and fear of it may vary across country and culture to a greater or lesser extent (Dryhurst et al. 2020). For instance, in the US, some people perceive it as no more serious than the common flu, whereas in China people make sense of COVID-19 as a serious disease that threatens their health and may have devastating consequences on the society at large. Though there are cultural differences across countries in terms of understanding the impact of COVID-19 on public health, it is also important to understand the political landscape of the country that would ultimately shape the attitude and influence the actions of the population toward it (Devine et al. 2020). In China, an authoritarian political system has shaped powerful narratives surrounding COVID-19 and influenced people's understanding and attitudes toward it. It is constructed as a public health risk of the highest level. Thus, in this chapter – as a result of strong governmentality – risk is perceived as a product of a series of governing techniques imposed on people (Ericson 1997). "Governmentality", as defined by Foucault, refers to a wide range of control techniques wielded by authorities to produce common knowledge and certain social actors (Foucault 1976).

In China, the rigorous measures put in place to control individual movements and behavior in order to eliminate COVID-19 have resulted in a heightened level of risk and individualized fear among individuals and communal fear of the local community as well as the workforce that were directly involved in the management and elimination of the COVID-19 transmission.

In five rounds of online surveys carried out by the Institute of Sociology, Chinese Academy of Social Sciences from January 24 to February 10, 2020, around 69.9% to 82% paid close attention to the COVID-19 pandemic and 17% to 27.8% paid relative attention to it. Around half of those surveyed felt that the virus might spread to their community (IOS CASS 2020).[6] Individuals and community considered the COVID-19 pandemic as a high-risk illness affecting the individual self and the local community, and it resulted in fear. There was individualized fear as individuals were afraid that they or their family members would become seriously ill or even face death when they were infected with the virus. At the community level, there was fear that individuals and their community would be implicated and blamed for a lockdown and movement restriction should they test positive. Government officials and workers also experienced heightened level of fear should there be positive COVID-19 cases appearing in their community as they would be blamed for not rigorously implementing the policies and actions within the grid community of their care. As mentioned earlier, there was intense surveillance on the performance of these workers to ensure that the community attained zero COVID-19 transmission. And failure would be the responsibility of those frontline workers and the local government officials.

When considering COVID-19 fears and risks, one must also consider the role played by trust. The success or failure of implementing the policies, strategies and actions to curb COVID-19 infection had also impacted the way individuals negotiated their level of trust and distrust of the various governmental and non-governmental agencies (Devine et al. 2020). During the initial COVID-19 outbreak, the chaotic handling of the COVID-19 situation led to a trust deficit among the Chinese citizens toward the central, provincial and local governments. There are different forms of trust. From a micro-substantive perspective, it may refer to rational, cognitive or affective responses of individuals in the face of uncertainties and actions taken to cope with it. It could also be divided into interpersonal trust and system trust. System trust takes abstract systems as its object, such as trust in the political system, expert system or other systems. System trust is an essential type of trust in a modern society that has developed increased complexities of social realities going beyond individuals' immediate experience (Beck 1992; Giddens 1991). Luhmann conceptualized trust as a mechanism for the reduction of complexities that "has absorbed certain functions and attributes of familiarity (and therefore really stands beyond personally generated trust or distrust)" (Luhmann 1979, 64). Trust is not simply a psychological state of mind but also can be a risk-taking action (Luhmann 1979; Das and Teng 2004).

According to Luhmann, trust is controlled "by subjective processes whereby experience is processed and simplified" (Luhmann 1979, 82). It involves a process of generalization of objects or events, either positive or negative, wherein people engage with information and experience selectively and subjectively. System trust goes beyond a "naïve" experience of the everyday world and is based on a conscious awareness that everything is arranged or produced (Luhmann 1979). In this way, governmentality forces entered the process of trust construction by exerting a wide array of discursive governing techniques that shape people's perception of risk and fear, their knowledge on COVID-19 as well as their concept of system functions. In a time of crisis such as the COVID-19 pandemic, the situation is undergoing constant changes and as a response, trust's subjective basis, both in cognitive and emotional senses, is also subjected to negotiation and contestation as a result of people's reflective engagement with COVID-19 transmission and the enforcement of government-directed COVID-19 policy. As we illustrated below, trust or distrust is non-static but is a continuously changed feature during the pandemic. As such, the initial pandemic outbreak is instrumental in shaping people's distrust of the governmental responses to the virus containment.

COVID-19, as a novel coronavirus, first drew public attention in China in conjunction with vehement criticism of the Wuhan government for its handling of the outbreak. When COVID-19 was first spotted in the Wuhan Huanan Sea Food Market in late 2019, the municipal government had chosen to downplay its severity. By the time China's top infectious disease expert reported to the central government, COVID-19 had already spread into the Wuhan city community. As COVID-19 was an unknown infectious virus and its rapid transmission had created anger and fear in both the affected community and the wider Chinese society, the population took to social media, such as WeChat, to vent their fear and anger. Public outrage reached a climax as seen from the intense communications and discontentment found on WeChat, Sina Weibo and others Chinese digital platforms when the whistleblower Dr. Li Wenliang died of COVID-19. As early as December 2019, Dr. Li, an ophthalmologist in Wuhan Central Hospital, shared with his friends a confidential report on novel coronavirus and warned them to keep away from Huanan Sea Food Market. Subsequently, the report was circulated on social media which resulted in Li being summoned and admonished by the Wuhan police for spreading false information. To the general public, Dr. Li Wenliang's incident reflected the highhandedness of the Chinese state in dealing with the emergent public health issue by suppressing information and the unwillingness to listen to public opinion as attested by the punishment of Dr. Li Wenliang. In Communist China today, COVID-19 remains a sensitive issue and any negative reports would be suppressed and taken off the digital media platforms immediately. This is especially so for reports on the inability and shortcomings of the government in dealing with this public health issue. As the COVID-19 infection spread across the country and with mounting public criticisms, the central government reacted that led to the withdrawal of the admonishment of Dr. Li and punished the relevant officers at the municipal level (*Renmin Ribao*, February 7, 2020 https://share.gmw.cn/politics/2020-02/07/content_33534903.htm, accessed January 27, 2022).

The incident of Dr. Li opened a Pandora's box that revealed a high level of public distrust of not only the Wuhan municipal government but also other governmental agencies. In another case, public suspicion and distrust were directed toward China's expert system. In late January 2020, the Chinese Centre for

Disease Control and Prevention (CDC) and its director, Gao Fu, drew heated discussions and criticism from the public because of an academic publication on China's COVID-19 situation in the *New England Journal of Medicine*. The author Gao drew a conclusion in the article that COVID-19 had spread into to the Wuhan community as early as December 2019. During the outbreak, the public blamed the Wuhan authorities for the late warning and slow response. The publication by Gao, who was a top official expert, seemed to confirm public suspicion that China's medical authority was also engaged in COVID-19 information cover-up. The public used social media to express their suspicion that the CDC's experts intentionally kept data and information away from the public's eyes for the purpose of publication and their own career advancement. In response to this criticism, the medical experts publicly clarified that the conclusion of the published article was derived using a scientific model from existing data on COVID-19 cases. Furthermore, a mainstream media report claimed that the CDC, although affiliated with the central government, was not tasked as the authority to release information of the COVID-19 pandemic to the public. Their role was restricted to carry out research and provide advice to the government health department (Sina Finance, January 31, 2020 https://finance.sina.cn/2020-01-31/detail-iimxyqvy9283390.d.html, accessed November 15, 2021).

Debates revolving around Dr. Li Wenliang and CDC experts reflected how the public viewed the pandemic crisis as one of uncertainty, fear and risk. Given the scant information relating to COVID-19 and the chaotic scenes reported in the media, it was not surprising that the public laid blame on the government, government bureaucracy and the specialized expert system for their ineptness in a COVID-19 laden uncertain environment where public fear, anxiety and distrust were high.

According to Luhmann, trust or distrust is a reduction of complexity in coping with uncertainty and it is also a tacit agreement to take controllable risks. The outbreak of COVID-19 and lack of knowledge on it generated a new complexity and uncertainty that the public had to grapple with, resulting in the re-activation of a simplifying process to understand the situation and reconstruct meanings and truth based on a selective choice of information, knowledge and ideas. Thus, during the transition of trust/distrust, some events gained special relevance and predominance over others. In our case, the public blamed the slow response of Wuhan government for its failure to contain the virus in the first place. Likewise, the acquisition of scientific knowledge by CDC is usually not a topic of public interest. But during the early phase of the COVID-19 pandemic where COVID-19 information was scant; the public was in desperate need of information and truth to interpret what had happened around them and the actions that they had to comply with. Thus, the act of not sharing but instead publishing the COVID-19 related data and information in an academic journal had incurred the wrath of the public. Public criticism on this matter reflected a deep feeling of unease and further distrust. Thus, CDC's media response further muddled the already murky water and heightened distrust of the public. This issue reflected a paradoxical dilemma faced by modern science in dealing with scientific risk and the perception of risk

(Beck 1992). In the aforementioned case, scientists in the CDC sought scientific evidence to confirm the risk factor while emotions and perceptions governed how the public viewed social risk attached to COVID-19.

The lack of information on COVID-19 created not only uncertainty but also inability of the individuals to proactively deal with it. The following accounts further revealed how individuals struggled in dealing with the outbreak and that led to their distrust in the local governments. According to interviewee Yin,

> My children and I were in Beijing and visited the Forbidden City on 19th January, 2020. It was a crowded public place. The next day, I heard of this virus (COVID-19-sic) from a member on this trip. He was quite alert and took a quick response. He went to the pharmacy and bought masks and distributed them to us. But I had no sense at all and only asked for a few. Several days later, we flew to Shantou for the Spring festival. Messages on the virus went viral in the social media and it was then that I realized the situation was serious and might even get worse. I felt worried for having visited Beijing and the Forbidden City and got infuriated at the government's handling of the disease. I would not have arranged a trip to Beijing if I knew what had happened in Wuhan. At that time, I felt it was the government's cover-up and they hid the information that had led to the spread of the virus, so we connected the outbreak with Chernobyl accident in former Soviet Union.

In comparing the COVID-19 outbreak with the Chernobyl nuclear disaster, interviewee Yin indicated that the spread of COVID-19 virus was due to the lack of transparency and the inertial responses of China's rigid and oppressive authoritarian bureaucratic system. This blame assignment was similar to the criticism of the Wuhan government's treatment of Dr. Li Wenliang where the public also drawn upon the oppressive and rigid characteristics of China's authoritarian political system. In Luhmann's words,

> Familiarity is the precondition for trust as well as distrust, i.e. for every sort of commitment to a particular attitude toward the future. Hazardous as well as propitious outlooks requires a certain familiarity, a socially constructed typicality, so as to make it possible to accommodate oneself to the future in a trustful or distrustful manner.
>
> (1979, 22)

A social understanding of authoritarianism enabled the people to navigate through this hazardous moment of virus outbreak in order to simplify the newly emerged complexity, albeit in a negative sense that reinforced their distrust of the system.

The anger and fear felt by Yin were also the dominant social emotions prevailing in China during the COVID-19 outbreak. Feelings, though capricious, are also part of the "elementary mechanisms of complexity reduction" (Luhmann 1979, 89). It is done so by "settling preferences on one object, and accordingly at the same time establish internal possibilities of processing experiences" (Luhmann

1979, 89). In other words, emotions and feelings, with relevance to trust or distrust construction, are part of a mechanism that makes people target on one object in a non-transferable manner so as to exclude other possibilities of explanation and understanding. Thus, when fear and anger are ignited socially, they reinforce people's distrust in the authorities and systems.

Likewise, there was also heightened public suspicion that government officials concealed official COVID-19 information about the Wuhan outbreak. According to interviewee Wang, who had a network of friends living overseas, she would source and trust COVID-19 information from her overseas friends rather than those provided by the Chinese government. She said: "my sister in U.S.A told me China must have tens of thousands of more confirmed cases than had been released. I guess she might be right. At least, Hubei's data seem to be downplayed by the government". Likewise, informant Ling also sought alternative source of information by watching Hong Kong TV channels. From this external source of information, she concluded that that data on COVID-19 cases in Hubei were not reliable. Misinformation is a common phenomenon during a pandemic (Roozenbeek et al. 2020). This is especially so in China where withholding and selected dissemination of information were perceived by the public as closely related to institutionalized censorship and intentional disguise and manipulation by the government in order that the Communist state has full control of the COVID-19 situation.

In this sense, mounting distrust of the government bureaucracies and expert system during the COVID-19 outbreak was reflected in the public narratives of authoritarian weakness, bureaucratic rigidity, information scarcity and misinformation. Coupled with the prevailing emotions of fear and anger, it pointed to a subjective process of generalization of information and ideas that help the public to cope and navigate this hazardous complex public health landscape posed by the fast-changing nature of the COVID-19 pandemic.

Turning the corner: the transition to multi-level trust

Public discontent and distrust of the government's response to the COVID-19 had reached a high point by 2020. The central government acted to calm the heart of the general public through new strategies and bringing in Zhong Nanshan, a health specialist who became known as the COVID-19 expert and acted as the COVID-19 pandemic's spokesperson. Through various strategies and the installation of Zhong as the COVID-19 expert, COVID-19 infection rates were brought down rapidly and ultimately contained with the zero-infection goal in sight. As China's COVID-19 infection was brought under control, there was also a corresponding increase in the level of trust toward the government where increasing number of people in the public acknowledged the effectiveness of the new strategies of COVID-19 containment and trust in Zhong's COVID-19 expertise. Here, we see a transition from distrust to trust among the Chinese public.

To understand this transition, we turned to Luhmann who argued that a transition between trust and distrust entails a threshold: on the one hand, it opens up more possibilities, and on the other hand, "simplifying processes of reduction, of orientation toward a few prominent key experiences, come into play. Objects and events, which appear to have value as indicator, gain special relevance, and control the interpretation of other situations" (Luhmann 1979, 83). In China, the transition was facilitated by a series of swift actions and propaganda campaigns taken by the central government, along with the speedy policy implementation at the community level. This constituted a threshold at which there was a change of social attitudes from one of distrust to trust.

The magnitude of the COVID-19 pandemic has led to large public discontent that could create social unrest, social dysfunction and social fragmentation. As such, the central government, under President Xi Jinping, took control and devised new strategies in quick response to public discontent. There was "an overall public-led agenda process, with government responding to both issues and emotions among the public in China" (Dai et al. 2021, 172). As mentioned above, the case of Dr. Li Wenliang demonstrated the central government's desire to gain an upper hand of the situation and hence took control and punished the Wuhan officials to quench the intense public anger.

At the same time, it installed Zhong Nanshan, a top respiratory expert in China as the COVID-19 pandemic spokesperson to assure the public of their full control over the pandemic situation and to regain the public trust. Zhong Nanshan earned his fame and popularity from his contribution to the management of the SARS outbreak in 2003. He was also the first medical expert to publicly confirm the human transmission of COVID-19 and the virus spread in Wuhan (*Beijing Daily*, January 21, 2020, https://news.sina.com.cn/o/2020-01-21/doc-iihnzhha3791299.shtml, accessed January 27, 2022). As such, he was viewed in the social media and mainstream press as an independent medical expert who dared to contradict the government authority. Because of his medical expertise and his perceived independence, he was recruited to advise on the strategies to combat the COVID-19 situation and his assessments and quarantine recommendation were adopted by the central and provincial governments. This included a nationwide lockdown in early 2020. Likewise, his recommendation of mask wearing and social distancing became the central government policy. He became the official voice both within China and outside and appeared regularly in China's official news press. Global Times, China's official English language news outlets for foreign audiences, reported one comment made by Zhong emphasized that "China has adopted a right path since the COVID-19 outbreak by making an all-out effort to curb the spread of the virus, and prevention-centered strategy will continue to dominate" (*Global Times*, March 10, 2021, https://www.globaltimes.cn/page/202110/1235607.shtml, accessed January 27, 2022). Through the incorporation of Zhong as the scientific and medical expert and using him as mouthpiece of its propaganda campaign and control, the central government is seeking to lure the public back to support its COVID-19 actions and regain their trust.

Another policy adopted was the strict lockdown when a COVID-19 cluster emerged and spread. From late January to April in 2020, there was a general lockdown that affected movement of people, especially during the lunar Chinese New

Year period. Social activities were suspended, and families and communities were isolated from each other, leading to a state of limbo. It was a dramatic experience and the sight of empty streets that was once lively created shockwaves among its population. However, according to informant Lin, she stated that although she got shocked to see once lively streets had gone completely empty, she nevertheless felt well protected by such a drastic strategy as the virus could not spread in her neighborhood. This is in sharp contrast to some other countries such as Italy where people perceived government containment measures during the outbreak as not useful (Vai et al. 2020). During strict lockdown, people could not go about their normal everyday life activities and a state of liminality prevailed. This lockdown constituted a second threshold in Luhmann's term wherein positive perception and reception of COVID-19 policy started to gain dominance. When lockdown came to an end in late April and the virus was successfully contained in China, people expressed high level of satisfaction and trust in the Chinese governments. A large-scale online survey conducted in late April 2020 to examine Chinese citizen's satisfaction and trust in China's COVID-19 policy showed the following results. When asked how their trust in the national and local levels of government had changed, 49.2% of respondents said more trusting in the national government since the outbreak and around 30% said to have more trust in local governments (Wu et al. 2021).

Among the participants interviewed, many changed their views from an initial distrust to trust and supportive of the government actions. One such person is Yin, who initially compared the virus spread with the Chernobyl accident, but later changed her opinion:

> I was a bit emotional at the start because COVID-19 might threaten my family. Now I tend to think the government was facing a very complex situation at the beginning and had to make a balance between COVID-19 containment and other issues.

Another participant, Zhou, explained that:

> At the outset, the virus hit Wuhan so unexpectedly that I think the government got lost. They did not know what the virus was and how it spread. During the spring festival period, Wuhan's medical emergency system was ill-prepared and lacked vigilance to tackle the virus. But the government had made quick and sensible responses to cope with it. The lockdown was timely and effective. There is no perfect person, so is the country. A country is composed of numerous individuals. As long as it protects the majority's life, I think it will gain trust from people.

According to Zhi:

> Authoritarian control has many weaknesses, but it is usually very effective to achieve a determined goal especially in a state of emergency such as COVID-19 outbreak. China had done a good job in containing the virus.

Likewise, Ling who was suspicious of government data during the outbreak, had a change of heart and dismissed a discussion on an unreported COVID-19 case among her friends. She said:

> I think it is just a rumor. I now tend to believe in the official data. We have a big retail store in IBC, the building where two COVID-19 cases were spotted recently. In no time we received a notice to suspend all business and to receive nucleic acid tests. And just within a few days, all people working in this building were tested three times, and the fourth test is about to come. We talked to staff in the workstation. They said they would rather be prudent and keep vigilant. No one could bear the consequences of cover-up or neglecting assigned COVID-19 duty now. Under such a strict regulation on officials, nobody in governments would dare to engage in cover up any more, I guess. Many messages about newly unreported COVID-19 cases are just rumors.

When COVID-19 spread worldwide and some countries such as the US were badly hit by it, interviewee Bin made this comparison and spoke highly of the mainland Chinese government's COVID-19 policy:

> I feel lucky in China. How other countries are affected by COVID-19! I do not believe those tenets of individualism. I think people live in groups. For example, wearing a mask, you are protecting yourself as well as others. Society cannot sustain without a government. If there was no governance, society would become like scattered sands. In terms of China's COVID-19 prevention, government policy is altruism. China really does a good job. Economy is recovering and we could live our normal life.

With the successful containment of the COVID-19 virus along with the propaganda and punitive measures, there was a visible change of public attitude from that of distrust to trust in Chinese government's handling of the pandemic. Authoritarianism that enabled strong control and enforcement power was previously cited as a cause of the spread of COVID-19 infection, but now perceived as conducive to controlling the virus spread. To the mainland Chinese who were brought up with Communist ideology, most have regarded authoritarian rule and high compliance as a way of life and they do not question it. Even among the educated and western-educated elite, authoritarianism as an ideology is not a fixed negative concept. Its use is utilitarian and as long as it is beneficial to the individual and his/her family, it is accepted. The Chinese public, influenced by the life-long Communist ideology, massive propaganda campaigns and goaded by the Chinese government, together with a high level of collective consciousness and compliance, has also started articulating the superiority of the values of collectivism in contrast to western individualism to frame China's COVID-19 containment success. Such comparison acted as "symbolic fixing of outcomes" (Luhmann 1979, 29) and contributed to trust building and represented the individual's cognitive negotiation of meanings and their subjective engagement with COVID-19 governance and control.

Reassessing trust in China's zero-transmission policy

Across the world, many countries have achieved a high vaccination rate to shift their policies to one of coexistence with COVID-19, as they moved toward the "endemic phase". With the risk of COVID-19 infection continuing for over two years, China's zero-transmission strategy started facing challenges, especially when small community clusters of Delta and Omicron variant cases were detected in late 2021. China reinstated the lockdown policy and mass nucleic acid testing of the whole community whenever a person or two in the community tested positive. This has led to pandemic fatigue and a sense of helplessness among the public. Lockdown, once perceived as protective, has turned out to be disruptive. However, any contrasting opinion would not be tolerated in a tightly controlled China. For example, when another popular doctor in Shanghai Huashan Hospital, Zhang Wenhong, suggested a relaxation of the COVID-19 control in 2021, he was instantly excoriated online. Likewise, official media also echoed such criticism from the mouth of a former health minister (Renmin Ribao, July 8, 2021 https://www.163.com/dy/article/GH430G350514WIJ2.html, accessed January 21, 2022).

A sense of helplessness has given way to grievance and dissatisfaction as well as fear and doubt. According to Song:

> Each time when I receive a nucleic test, I am quite worried for having contracted the virus because that equals to a sentence of social death. My neighbors would be quarantined because of me; my son's school may face a sudden lockdown etc. That makes me worried and feared more than contracting COVID-19. I still trust the central government as well as management in big cities such as Beijing, Shanghai and Shenzhen, but not other cities. China's preventive policy does not have big problems and it is effective and responsive. The result of COVID-19 control is satisfactory to me, but sometimes I still doubt if there are soft but effective methods to achieve the same result.

As the pandemic dragged on and with no change of policy in sight, the Chinese with full vaccination status in their local community became worried and fearful, not of contracting the virus but social ostracism they would face should they contracted COVID-19. At the same time, individuals were beginning to differentiate between different levels of trust that they bestowed on the central, provincial and local governments. Participant Zhou said:

> The highest administrative level, the central government provides directives and guidance. Local government set up concrete measures in accordance with it. But the actual implementation of COVID-19 policy is affected by local governments' management competency, economic scale, their ability to

> pool resources etc. First tier cities are more likely to be flexible and humanized in implementing COVID-19 policy while some under-developed regions would follow a very rigid and harsh method and impose uniformity in actual implementation of COVID-19 policy. As for the trust, I trust more in the central government but less in lower level governments' implementation. But overall, as long as it protects the majority's life, it will gain my trust to the greatest extent.

Another interviewee, Yin, mentioned that she trusted the central government more:

> I trust the central government. I think that is a big trust. As for trust in local government and community, this is a small trust, a realization of big trust in everyday life. To me, big trust (in central government) is the precondition for small trust.

The differentiation of levels of trust in China's COVID-19 control is one where social trust was subordinate to system trust. The overall control has left little space for local community to take independent action and response. Trust has been counteracted with punitive fear of non-compliance and social stigmatization. Under this situation, it is reflective of the extent to which governmentality of the state has penetrated into the local community that manifested itself as both suppressive power as well as productive power. These two powers were capable of shaping people's mind, knowledge and perception that ultimately influenced the types of behavior and actions to attain individual compliance during this period of COVID-19 pandemic. While mass compliance had been the key, there were also small groups of individuals who defied the regulatory control such as by refusing to wear a mask, maintain social distancing or follow quarantine rules – usually leading to official punishment and even social condemnation.[7]

Trust in China during the COVID-19 pandemic could be characterized in the following manner: a high level of trust placed on the central government for the overall directives and planning on the formulation of COVID-19 policy and a low level of trust placed on the governments and officials at local levels pertaining to the implementation and enforcement of COVID-19 policies laid down by the central government. In understanding trust formation, it enabled us to understand the work of China's authoritarian political system where power delegated downstream also brought along local responsibility. Thus, inability to control the spread of the COVID-19 infection or public discontent would be the responsibility of the local governments and local officials. Such a system absolved the central government from overall responsibility of failures. As such, China's multi-level governance placed central authority above reproach while provincial, municipal, county and local governments were held accountable for the success and failure of policy implementation and actions. Under such a pyramidal political system, central government has established a leverage to manipulate public opinion where high-level trust was placed in the central government by the public while local governments were less trusted.

Conclusion

In conclusion, this chapter has demonstrated that China, as a Communist state with an authoritarian system of governance, has been able to eliminate and slow down the COVID-19 transmission because of the unified approach directed from the central government downwards to the local community. By moderating the dissenting voices in the public, the central government established a multi-level COVID-19 governance framework and activated the grid governance system to mobilize ground officials to act on policies and strategies and implemented acts to curb the spread of COVID-19 in the local community. From the initial chaotic start to a systematic approach of track and trace, social distancing, personal hygiene, reports, semi-lockdowns, lockdowns and quarantines, China has managed to stop the COVID-19 spread in its track.

Correspondingly, constant campaigns and information released by the central, provincial, municipal and local governments were attempts to direct the public toward the success of the policies and strategies. At the same time, through media, it constantly compared its success with the messy outbreaks and high rate of daily infections elsewhere, the non-compliance of the western public with mask wearing, social distancing and vaccination in the western parts of the world. All these have swung public opinion from one of fear and distrust to one of trust, where the public differentiated between the level of trust between the central government, provincial and local governments.

COVID-19 with its changing variants continued to impact on all communities and China is not immune to it. At the beginning of 2022, half of China has COVID-19 cases emerging and China continued its policy of semi-lockdown and restricted movements of its people. The question that emerged in the minds of its people is "when will this end?" and the resignation that they would still have to comply with the strict policies and restricted movements for the good of the country as they waited for the complete elimination of the COVID-19 pandemic.

Postscript

After achieving zero COVID-19 for two years, toward the end of 2021, there was a flare up of COVID-19 cases in different parts of China. Following the initial Xian outbreak, it spread to Shenzhen, Guangzhou, Shanghai and Beijing. Each day, there were over 30 to 40 districts throughout China that had cases of COVID-19 infection. China continued its "dynamic zero COVID-19 policy" and districts infected were subjected to lockdowns. As of May 2022, all provinces adopted stringent COVID-19 policy, performing mass nucleic acid testing once every two or three days, restricting movements and initiating lockdowns. This has led to stress, fear and uncertainty that ultimately led to an increase in a high level of policy distrust and the COVID-19 management and governance. This is especially so because while other countries around the world were opening up and returning to normalcy, China was adopting a reverse policy of lockdown again.

Fear, stress and distrust had led to residents taking to social media to vent their anger and frustration. However, the long arm of the state immediately took action to scrub clean any negative postings online. Despite this, the voices of the citizens residing in various cities continued to appear on social media and use it to their full advantage for communication with each other and to the general public.

For China, the management and governance of COVID-19 is a highly centralized affair and power ultimately rests with the central government. Governments at decentralized levels must carry out the directives from the central government downwards. Deviations from this is not tolerated and would be brought into alignment. The return to normalcy could only be realized if the central government removed its "dynamic zero policy" and accepted the idea of mutual coexistence with the COVID-19 virus and treated it as an endemic rather than a pandemic.

Notes

1 Khun Eng Kuah, first and corresponding author.
2 Cohen, J. (February 19, 2020). "Scientists 'strongly condemn' rumors and conspiracy theories about origin of coronavirus outbreak. A statement in the Lancet assails misinformation about the possibility that COVID-19 came from a lab in Wuhan, China". (https://www.science.org/content/article/scientists-strongly-condemn-rumors-and-conspiracy-theories-about-origin-coronavirus), accessed January 23, 2022.
3 In Chinese *wang ge hua zhili* (网格化治理).
4 Danwei community in Chinese is *danwei shequ* (单位社区), street residential community in Chinese is *jieju shequ* (街居社区) and commercial housing community in Chinese is *shangpinfang shequ* (商品房社区).
5 For example, a total of 15 officials in Nanjing were punished for ineffective epidemic control and prevention in 2021. *Global Times*, August 7, 2021, https://www.globaltimes.cn/page/202108/1230812.shtml, accessed January 26, 2022.
6 The first round of survey was conducted from January 24 to January 25, 2020; the second round was from January 25 to 29, 2020; the third round was from January 29 to February 2, 2020; the fourth round was from February 2 to February 6, 2020 and the fifth round was from February 7 to February 10, 2020. In these five rounds of survey,79.1%, 81.6%, 81.6%, 82% and 69.9% paid close attention to COVID-19, respectively, while 20.1%, 18%, 17.3%, 17.0% and 27.8% paid relative attention to it.
7 For example, a returning overseas student jumped the bus to escape check and quarantine, who faced both official and social condemnation. *Qingdao News*, March 30, 2020, https://baijiahao.baidu.com/s?id=1662558644395983382&wfr=spider&for=pc, accessed January 27, 2022.

References

Beck, Ulrich. 1992. *Risk Society: Towards a New Modernity*. London: Sage.

Dai, Yixin, Yuejiang Li, Chao-Yo Cheng, Hong Zhao and Tianguang Meng. 2021. "Government-Led or Public-Led? Chinese Policy Agenda Setting during the COVID-19 Pandemic." *Journal of Comparative Policy Analysis: Research and Practice*, 23(2): 157–175. DOI:10.1080/13876988.2021.1878887.

Das, T. K. and Bing-Sheng Teng. 2004. "The Risk-Based View of Trust: A Conceptual Framework." *Journal of Business and Psychology*, 19 (1):85–116.

Devine, Daniel, Jennifer Gaskell, Will Jennings and Gerry Stoker. 2020. "Trust and the Coronavirus Pandemic: "What are the Consequences of and for Trust? An Early Review of the Literature." *Political Studies Review*, 2020:1–12. DOI:10.1177/1478929920948684.

Douglas, Mary. 1992. *Risk and Blame: Essays in Cultural Theory*. London; New York: Routledge.

Dryhurst, Sarah, Claudia R. Schneider, John Kerr, Alexandra L.J. Freeman, Gabriel Recchia, Anne Marthe van der Bles, David Spiegelhalter and Sander van der Linden. 2020. "Risk Perceptions of COVID-19 around the World." *Journal of Risk Research*, 23:7–8, 994–1006. DOI:10.1080/13699877.2020.1758193.

Ericson, Richard Victor. 1997. *Policing the Risk Society*. Oxford: Oxford University Press.

Foucault, Michel. 1976. "Two Lectures" in *Critique and Power: Recasting the Foucault/Habermas Debate*, edited by Kelly, Michael. 1994. Massachusetts; London: The MIT Press.

Giddens, Anthony. 1991. *The Consequences of Modernity*. Cambridge: Polity Press.

Giddens, Authony. 1998. *The Third Way: The renewal of Social Democracy*. Cambridge: Polity Press.

IOS (Institute of Sociology, Chinese Academy of Social Sciences). 2020. "The Evolution of Social Attitudes in Pandemic within 18 Days." http://css.cssn.cn/shxsw/swx_kycg/swx_yjbg/202002/t20200218_5090128.html (in Chinese), accessed 28/1/2022.

Li, Peilin. 2020. "Grassroots Community Management in COVID-19." *Social Management*, 2020(12). http://www.sociology2010.cass.cn/xscg/zxwz/202101/t20210125_5247032.shtml (in Chinese).

Liu, Jun and Hui Zhao. 2021. "Privacy Lost: Appropriating Surveillance Technology in China's Fight Against COVID-19." *Business Horizons*, 2021(64):743–756. DOI: https://doi.org/10.1016/j.bushor.2021.07.004

Liu, Zhilin, Jing Guo, Wei Zhong and Tianhan Gui. 2021. "Multi-Level Governance, Policy Coordination and Subnational Responses to COVID-19: Comparing China and the US." *Journal of Comparative Policy Analysis: Research and Practice*, 23(2):204–218. DOI:10.1080/13876988.2021.1873703.

Luhmann, Niklas. 1979. *Trust and Power*. Chichester: Wiley.

Roozenbeek, Jon, Claudia R. Schneider, Sarah Dryhurst, John Kerr, Alexandra L. J. Freeman, Gabriel Recchia, Anne Marthe van der Bles and Sander van der Linden.2020. "Susceptibility to Misinformation about COVID-19 around the World." *Royal Society Open Science* 7:201199. DOI: http://dx.doi.org/10.1098/rsos.201199

Vai, Benedetta, Silvia Cazzetta, Davide Ghiglino, Lorenzo Parenti, Giacomo Saibene, Michelle Toti, Chiara Verga, Agnieszka Wykowska and Francesco Benedetti. 2020. "Risk Perception and Media in Shaping Protective Behaviors: Insights from the Early Phase of COVID-19 Italian Outbreak." *Frontiers in Psychology* 11:563426. DOI: 10.3389/fpsyg.2020.563426.

Wu, Cary, Zhilei Shi, Rima Wilkes, Jiaji Wu, Zhiwen Gong, Nengkun He, Zang Xiao et al. 2021. "Chinese Citizen Satisfaction with Government Performance during COVID-19." *Journal of Contemporary China*, 30(132):930–944. DOI: 10.1080/10670564.2021.1893558.

Zhu, Tianke, Xigang Zhu and Jian Jin. 2021. "Grid Governance in China under the COVID-19 Outbreak: Changing Neighhorhood Governance." *Sustainability* 13(13):7089. DOI: https://doi.org/10.3390/su13137089

5 COVID-19 responses of displaced slum dwellers in Delhi

Who to trust and rely on in times of sanitary and economic crisis?

Véronique Dupont[1] *and M. M. Shankare Gowda*

Introduction

On March 24, 2020, at 20.00, with 519 confirmed COVID-19 cases recorded for the entire country,[2] the Indian prime minister announced a national lockdown with four hours' notice. The lockdown was extended three consecutive times and lasted 68 days, followed by a gradual lifting of restrictions. The abrupt cessation of economic activities had the hardest impact on the multitude of low-income, informally employed and self-employed workers (Kesar et al. 2020; Naik 2020; Unni 2020). The urban poor living in substandard and overcrowded settlements found it almost impossible to follow sanitary and social distancing norms (Auerbach and Thachil 2021; Bercegol et al. 2020; Downs-Tepper, Krishna and Rains 2022). These two categories of population largely overlap in cities, compounding their vulnerability during the pandemic. Similar situations that exacerbated precariousness and socioeconomic inequalities were observed in other countries (De Groot and Lemanski 2021; Wilkinson et al. 2020). This chapter considers such an affected group – the former residents of a large slum settlement in Delhi – who were evicted from their previous habitat a few years ago, mostly now resettled in a transit camp and are still awaiting their final rehabilitation. We address in this case study the responses of local communities to the first COVID-19 wave and explore the issues of risk and trust in this period of crisis and challenging socio-spatial context. It is however important to situate the risk and fear of the disease in the broader context of the multiple risks faced by the urban poor living in hazardous environments and unsanitary squatter settlements (Wratten 1995), including permanent eviction threat as already experienced by the slum dwellers in our case study. During the lockdown, and as confirmed by several of our respondents and reported in the media (Mander 2020), the bigger risk and highest concern for the urban poor who lost their access to livelihoods was dying of hunger, not of COVID.

In his addresses to the nation about the lockdown and its extensions, the Indian prime minister called upon civil society organizations and citizens' solidarity to mitigate the poor's hardships (Hebbar 2020; *Economic Times* 2020a), thereby largely discharging the state of its responsibility in the matter. Although the Union finance minister announced some relief packages (*Economic Times* 2020b),[3] these

DOI: 10.4324/9781003291220-5

were considered grossly insufficient, deceptive and poorly implemented, therefore not reaching the intended beneficiaries (Azim Premji University 2020; HLRN 2020; Khera and Somanchi 2020; Unni 2020). Indeed, civil society played a key role in responding to the lockdown-induced crisis in Indian cities (Bercegol et al. 2020; Naik 2020), including in our case study, and as observed in other countries (Duque Franco et al. 2020).

To investigate the issue of trust, in line with Giddens (1990) and Luhmann (1979), we differentiate two types of trust: a system-based trust, placed in the system or institution, and an interpersonal trust, negotiated between individuals. This calls for considering the contextual factors at different levels, from the national to the local. We further examine to what extent Gidden's (1990) conception of "modernity", wherein trust is no longer placed in a person but in theoretically functioning "abstract systems", may apply in the pandemic context to the studied communities. Focusing on system-based trust, Spire (2020) further distinguishes a more abstract "symbolic confidence" that is "the belief in the legitimacy of the institution" (Spire 2020: 39 – our translation), from a "practical trust" in institutions, resulting from the accumulated practical experiences with specific institutions (Spire, 2020), which may change an *a priori* abstract opinion. By factoring in this dynamic dimension of trust, we better understand the distrust entrenched in most of our respondents of certain state institutions as well as some of their seemingly contradictory appreciations of the government measures during India's prolonged lockdown. Nooteboom (2007) underlined another interesting distinction between "trust in competence (ability to conform to expectations) and trust in intention (to perform in good faith according to the best of competence)" (Nooteboom 2007: 35). He further highlighted two dimensions of the latter: "commitment, i.e. attention to possible mishaps, and absence of opportunism" (Nooteboom 2007). We apply such distinctions to better qualify the interpersonal relationships of (dis)trust among members of the studied communities.

This chapter focuses on a large cluster of displaced slum dwellers in Delhi, most of whom have been temporarily resettled in a transit camp. "Who to trust and to rely on in times of sanitary and economic crisis" is the ultimate question we address, one which can be broken down in the following sub-questions. What do people's reactions to the government measures reveal about their trust in state institutions? Has fear of the virus engendered interpersonal mistrust among people? What do communities' responses tell us about the foundation of interpersonal trust and solidarity networks? Has the crisis essentially confirmed traditional solidarities based on family, caste and religion? Or has it allowed the emergence of new solidarity networks? To answer these questions, we need first to introduce the local setup – Kathputli Colony – and appraise the major impacts of the lockdown. Next, when examining the communities' responses, we distinguish between the coping strategies devised at the household level and the relief initiatives at the settlement level, referring also to the government relief schemes and to the role of non-governmental organizations (NGOs). Following this assessment, we consider the sanitary and economic crisis as a pointer, revealing relationships of trust – or mistrust – among the various players involved in this crisis and in its mitigation, including the residents themselves, external actors (NGOs, individual benefactors, local politicians) and institutions at different levels. With reference to the prime minister's appeal to civil society organizations, we notably question the level of trust that people place in these organizations versus in the state institutions. Our source of data and the methodology used are presented after the local setup.

Introducing the case study: the displaced residents of Kathputli Colony in Delhi

The contextualization of the settlement is essential for understanding its residents' relationship to public action, as well as the breeding ground of interpersonal (mis)trust.

A demolished informal settlement

In 2017, Kathputli Colony was an informal settlement of around 18,000 people, comprising a number of distinct communities differentiated mainly along lines of regional origin but also by caste, religious affiliation and occupation. The dominant social group is a community of folk artists and craftsmen from Rajasthan who were the first settlers in the late 1960s.[4] Social segmentation resulting from different migration flows translated into spatial segregation, with distinct sections of the settlement corresponding to different communities with their own local leader. It had become a heterogeneous settlement where varying housing conditions reflected socioeconomic disparities.

For the Delhi Development Authority (DDA), Kathputli Colony was an illegal slum occupying its valuable land in central Delhi (see Figure 5.1). The public urban planning agency targeted this settlement in 2008 to implement its first slum redevelopment project under a public–private partnership. The construction of the rehousing complex, several 14-story buildings, first required the demolition of the settlement and the relocation of its residents in a transit camp.

Retention of information and lack of transparency characterized the DDA mode of governance in the first phase of the project, raising anxiety and mistrust among the concerned residents. Thus, many key issues were unclear for several years, including the precise eligibility criteria to access a rehabilitation flat – and hence the list of eligible households, the financial conditionality and the occupancy status (Dupont et al. 2014). Two other issues fed the resistance of a large section of residents to this project and their ire against the public agency and the private developer who won the development contract. First, with no participatory approach, the rehousing project was conceived without considering the residents' needs. Second, the residents denounced a land grab at the expense of their own rights, as the land-sharing model of the project allocated 40% of the plot area for the developer's benefit.

However, another section of residents supported the rehabilitation project, considering it a good opportunity – or the only option – to improve their living

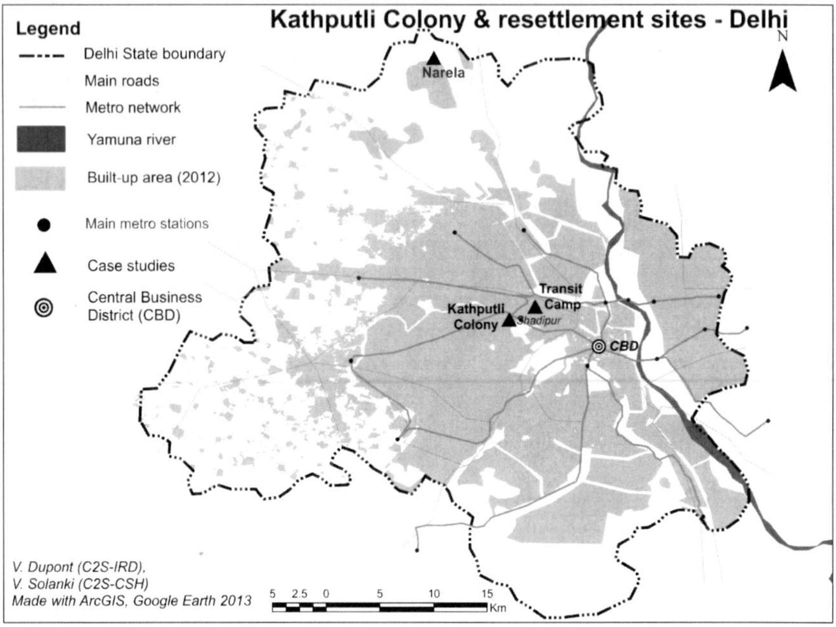

Figure 5.1 Kathputli Colony and the resettlement sites in the Delhi region.

conditions and secure their tenure. Some up-and-coming leaders further engaged in active negotiations with the DDA to obtain more guarantees. Eventually, a new line of fragmentation grew among the residents, between the pro-project group and the opponents of the project (Dupont and Gowda 2020). This dividing factor resulted in mutual mistrust, including within the same ethnic community, with long-lasting effects as observed during the pandemic.

The final and main evacuation drive occurred in late 2017, followed by the total demolition of the settlement. Nearly 13,500 people were forcibly evicted in three days by about 350 police forces backed by bulldozers. In the days, sometimes weeks, following the demolition, many families were shelterless, squatting near or on the rubble of the demolished site. Around 70% of the Kathputli Colony households were resettled in the transit camp while 12% of households were relocated to flats in a DDA housing scheme in the Narela township (see Figure 5.1). The remaining households were simply excluded from the rehabilitation program without compensation. Thus, the majority of the settlement's residents experienced the violent arm of the state and suffered from its callousness.

From the preliminary phase of the project implementation, up until the total demolition of the settlement, the residents were often disappointed in their deputies. The politicians were unable to defend the residents' interests and made false promises such as free flats, when in reality a consequential financial contribution is required of eligible households, likely to exclude poorer families.

This backdrop raises further research questions. How did these past experiences and disillusions influence the way the displaced residents relied – or not – on state institutions or on their elected representatives to provide them with aid during the pandemic? Through which lenses did they appraise the state's decisions and initiatives?

The resettlement sites: the transit camp and the Narela flats complex

The transit camp is located around three kilometers from the initial settlement on rocky wasteland. It houses 14,000 to 15,000 people in rows of 2,800 prefabricated one-room tenements of 12 sqm per household, irrespective of household size, with neither kitchen nor running water. Each row shares bathing facilities, and several toilet blocks are installed along the boundary walls of the camp. Shared outdoor taps supply drinking water, entailing long queues, especially in summer when water supply is limited and irregular. Despite a context of high-density settlement, cramped living conditions and poor sanitary arrangements, only a few mild cases of COVID-19 were reported in the camp in 2020.[5]

The households relocated to Narela accessed better housing conditions. They were allotted flats equivalent to the flats designed for the future in-situ rehousing complex (two-room flats of about 25 sqm with kitchen, attached bathroom and toilet). However, their relegation to the outskirts of the city – about 30 kilometers away from Kathputli Colony – entailed the disruption of earlier social and economic networks and difficult access to the city resources.

Like Kathputli Colony earlier, the relocation sites are home to an assemblage of multiple communities where previous lines of division have persisted. However, the resettlement process disrupted the previous socio-spatial organization (Dupont and Gowda 2021). In the transit camp, although some blocks are occupied exclusively or mainly by a single community, in many others different communities are mixed. In the Narela blocks of flats, community grouping is the exception, due to a random draw system of allotment. Many communities – even families – are split between the two relocation sites, not to mention the excluded households left to fend for themselves. Traditional local leaders have lost their authority and the trust of many residents who suspect them of having benefited from the developer's undue favors. Eventually, the forced displacement challenged to some extent old solidarities, with enduring consequences during the pandemic.

Additional factors have reinforced the residents' distrust and resentment of the DDA. As the construction of the rehousing complex is progressing very slowly, the stay in the transit camp is lasting much longer than initially announced. Furthermore, most residents did not get proper legal documents guaranteeing them a rehabilitation flat and are thus maintained under an insecure status.

Methodology

The first-hand data mobilized for this paper were collected through telephone interviews conducted between April and November 2020. The investigated issues were multidimensional impact of the lockdown, coping strategies devised at the household level, relief operations organized by various actors and their appreciation, solidarity networks, interpersonal trust and trust placed in different institutions during this crisis. Such a remote survey was made possible – and backed up – by extended research conducted since 2009 in Kathputli Colony and the relocation sites. Our long-lasting engagement with the residents of this settlement helped us build mutual understanding and trust-based relationships. It facilitated their acceptance of the telephone interviews and secured interpretation.

We adopted an actor-centered qualitative approach and applied a purposive sampling strategy to ensure the representation of the different communities. We first approached the contacts established during earlier fieldwork, including from a survey on the multidimensional effects of resettlement on the displaced families conducted in October–December 2019. The follow-up of previous respondents allowed us to better appraise the impact of the crisis on their socioeconomic condition. In addition, our network of contacts and recognized figures served as referrals to reach new respondents by phone. Our survey was positively received, as people appreciated the opportunity to explain their difficulties in this time of crisis. In return, they often expected help from the investigator.

Phone interviews had some advantages over the face-to-face interviews conducted earlier in the same communities. Mobile phones allowed respondents to talk more discreetly, with less interference from the people around them, and eventually more openly. This was especially valuable when interviewing women, who were able to express themselves freely without the customary male interference and influence. Additionally, in a space under surveillance like the transit camp, phone interviews enabled us to bypass the camp authorities and guards. We could not, however, confront the responses with direct observations – for instance, compliance with social distancing norms and masks.

We eventually carried out two series of phone interviews:

- With residents of the transit camp: 23 in-depth interviews (18 men, five women), including 11 with respondents interviewed during earlier surveys; and 16 shorter interviews (ten men, six women);
- With residents of the resettlement flats in Narela: seven in-depth interviews (five men interviewed earlier, two women); five shorter interviews with men; and additional interviews focusing on food distribution with seven protagonists.

In both locations, the respondents included former and up-and-coming community leaders, as well as relief work organizers. The mostly masculine leadership from Kathputli Colony explains the over-representation of men in our interviews.

Following the 2021 epidemic surge and lockdown, we conducted a second survey round to follow up on the impact and on the communities' responses. We carried out 40 in-depth interviews with residents from the same sample between June and August 2021, face-to-face in the transit camp, and mostly by telephone for Narela residents. Although this chapter focuses on the first COVID-19 wave, the 2021 investigations helped us consolidate – or nuance – our analysis.

The effects of the 2020 lockdown on livelihood

While the health effects of COVID-19 on the transit camp inhabitants were limited despite unfavorable housing conditions, the first lockdown with the abrupt suspension of economic activities and transport had a dramatic impact on their living conditions; it also affected those resettled in flats on the city outskirts. The effects were multiple, and some persisted after the lockdown was lifted. We highlight, hereafter, the major ones and distinguish between the immediate and more acute impact during the lockdown itself, and the longer-term effects observed up to six months (until November 2020, corresponding with our investigation period) after restriction measures were gradually relaxed. Our focus on economic consequences should not, however, overshadow the dramatic impact of school closure, forcing children to stay home in cramped rooms where living conditions made it difficult if not impossible for them to attend online classes even when these existed. This extended de-schooling – at least ten months – will likely have long-term consequences on the children's education and on early school dropouts.

The lockdown's direct impact

The people from Kathputli Colony are mostly either self-employed (folk artists and craftsmen, street vendors and shopkeepers, cycle-rickshaw pullers and auto-rickshaw drivers, etc.) or hold precarious or low-paid jobs with no social protection (factory workers, construction workers, domestic helpers, office or shop assistants, etc.). Overnight, all of them became unemployed with no source of income. Most employers did not comply with the central government's directive to pay their workers' wages during the lockdown. The lockdown was strictly enforced by the police, especially in informal settlements (Bercegol et al. 2020), and in the transit camp. The lack of income entailed food shortages and restrictions for the families. Nevertheless, compared to other urban low-income groups, especially migrant workers staying in rented accommodations,[6] the transit camp residents were in a better position since their lodging expenses – including electricity costs – were paid by the developer, in charge of the camp maintenance. In the Narela flats, the DDA pays housing and maintenance costs but not electricity, which increased the residents' financial difficulties in times of crisis.

Longer-term effects

When the national lockdown was lifted on June 1, the relaxation of restrictions was gradual. Economic activities restarted very slowly, partly due to the distancing norms imposed in workplaces limiting the number of workers at the same time, and partly because demand remained low. For the transit camp and Narela flats residents, unemployment or underemployment with casualization of work persisted for at least a couple of additional months. With factories and offices not functioning at full capacity, workers and employees resumed their work on alternative days at best, with a corresponding cut in salary. It took an even longer time for the performing artists to book shows, as the size of public and private gatherings was initially strictly limited. Auto-rickshaw drivers suffered from restrictions on the number of passengers allowed, as well as from the reluctance of people to travel in collective rickshaws because of COVID. In July, several women working as domestic helpers had not as yet been called back by their employers, due to the latter's contamination fears.

Altogether, lack of income during the lockdown, then irregular and reduced earnings in the following months led to the impoverishment and indebtedness of many families, as examined in the next section. Our findings corroborate the results of other surveys conducted during the lockdown, including in Delhi, showing that "food insecurity and economic vulnerability have increased to staggering proportions" (Azim Premji University 2020, 1; Downs-Tepper, Krishna and Rains 2022; Kesar et al. 2020).

Coping strategies and relief initiatives

What were the coping strategies devised at the household level to compensate for income shortfalls and job losses? Besides government relief measures, what were the collective or individual initiatives at the settlement level – or a section of it – by non-state actors to deal with this unprecedented crisis and respond first of all to food shortage? These are the main questions tackled in this section.

Coping strategies at the household level

With no income source, people started reducing their expenditure including on food, then began spending their savings – if any. Eventually, as the lockdown was extended, most had to borrow money. Depending on their family environment and occupational situation, some borrowed from relatives in town or in the village, others from work colleagues or from their employers or their contractors. Some regularly employed factory workers and domestic helpers got advance payment from their employers, based on trusting relationships. But for many, borrowing money meant resorting to moneylenders at usurious rates of 4% to 5% per month. Moneylenders from the transit camp were not more lenient with their fellow residents. Of particular concern is the practice of pawning valuables, especially women's gold ornaments. This practice is frequent in the Rajasthani community in times of crisis. However, given the extent of the COVID-19 induced crisis, and the high-interest rates, some respondents worried about their capacity to retrieve their jewelry. Other residents with no valuables pledged their official documents for allotment in the rehousing complex with the money lender. Theoretically, the DDA will not allot a flat to a non-enlisted household. Yet, in case of malpractices or difficulties reimbursing the loan, this practice seriously threatens the borrower's future housing prospects. From being a coping strategy and short-term solution to face income shortage, incurring secured debts may in the long run threaten the households' assets, as observed in rural areas during the lockdown (Guérin et al. 2020), and eventually aggravate impoverishment. Indeed, one year later, many families were debt-trapped and many could not yet retrieve their valuables.

To survive food insecurity during the lockdown, most households resorted to at least one type or other of external support, in the form of free distribution of rations or cooked meals organized by state and non-state actors inside or outside their settlement (the transit camp or the Narela flats complex). They also availed themselves – or attempted to – of government financial assistance schemes whenever eligible.

Before considering these various relief initiatives, we need to examine the household livelihood strategies in place while the containment measures were being gradually lifted starting June 1, 2020. As explained above, most workers could not resume their previous occupation straightaway. Since the priority was earning a living, the cost was accepting any kind of unskilled precarious work, even at the risk of one's health, as expressed by this former factory security guard who had still not been recalled by his employer by the end of June:

> People are ready to take any work for money, everybody is desperate for work, despite [COVID-19] cases increasing in Delhi, people are not bothered about it, for them now livelihood is more important than life.[7]
>
> (Authors' interview from the transit camp, June 25, 2020)

Unemployed men went to the labor market to be recruited by contractors as manual casual laborers, especially in the construction sector, including those, such as performing artists, who had never worked in this sector.

> So [since we are not getting any show] we are doing other menial jobs which is difficult and also hurts our professional dignity" (Authors' interview, October 2, 2020), complained a Rajasthani artist in the transit camp.

Yet, due to increased labor supply and therefore competition among workers, not everyone could find steady work. In some communities, unemployed people resorted to waste picking. Dire financial straits pushed several women into prostitution. Many others started begging for food with their children on the streets and in nearby better-off neighborhoods. Another coping strategy consisted in sending back the non-earning members (wife and/or children) to the home village once transport facilities resumed, which alleviated the household's expenses in times of employment crisis.

To sum up, the households' responses to the COVID-19-induced crisis show limited available fall-back options. Furthermore, these options increased people's dependence on moneylenders and on external assistance during the lockdown and pushed them into deteriorated employment opportunities or destitution in the following months. Increased indebtedness and precarious employment arrangements reflect the situation that prevailed in the country post-lockdown

(Abraham, Basole and Kesar 2021). In the next two sections we review the financial assistance schemes and various relief works the studied communities benefited from.

Government relief schemes in 2020

A number of relief measures were announced in 2020 by the central government at the national level and by the government of the National Capital Territory of Delhi (thereafter the Delhi government) to mitigate the adverse effects of the extended lockdown on the socioeconomically vulnerable groups (HLRN 2020). The central government launched the *Pradhan Mantri Garib Kalyan Yojana*[8] – the prime minister's food welfare scheme for the poor, as well as cash transfers. The communities in our study benefited from the following measures:

- Free supply of 5 kg of wheat grain or rice and 1 kg of pulse per adult and per month for three months (extended until November 2020) through the Public Distribution System in fair-price shops, to beneficiaries covered under the National Food Security Act, 2013, namely ration-card holders below the poverty line;
- Monthly cash transfers of 500 rupees for three months to women holding a *Jan-Dhan* bank account, also called a zero-deposit account under the National Mission for Financial Inclusion;[9]
- An *ex gratia* payment of 1,000 rupees to beneficiaries of national pension schemes for old age, widows and persons with disabilities;
- Free supply of cooking gas cylinders for three months through cash transfers to women beneficiaries of the *Pradhan Mantri Ujjwala Yojana*,[10] for households under the poverty line.

The Delhi government, in charge (like other state governments) of implementing the distribution of food rations, decreed complementary relief measures, including the following from which many residents of the transit camp and the Narela flats benefited:

- Free supply of additional quantities of food rations (50% more than the normal entitlement) for three months through government fair-price shops. Importantly, this scheme was extended to those without ration cards, basically to all needy households;
- Supplementary free ration kits, consisting of oil, sugar, salt, lentils or chickpeas and soap, distributed along with food grains, for three months;
- Free cooked meals provided in "hunger relief centers" – community kitchens usually housed in government schools – to all needy people unconditionally during the lockdown (till May 31, 2020);
- Advance payment of old-age pensions for three months;
- One-time compensation allowance of 5,000 rupees for electric and auto-rickshaw drivers, all of whom were banned from operating during the lockdown.

There is always a gap between the policy measures announced and their concrete implementation and outcome on the ground. Their impact is often impeded due to delays and dysfunctions (Azim Premji University 2020; HLRN 2020; Ngullie and Ansari 2021). It is important to note that the above-mentioned central government measures reached only the beneficiaries of prior national schemes, *de facto* leaving out many people. Moreover, people may not be well informed about conditions to access a specific scheme, for example, the free supply of gas cylinders. In the transit camp, most residents could not avail themselves of this facility, either because they were not registered with the *Ujjwala Yojana*, or because, while registered, they were uninformed of the modalities for applying.

Emergency food relief provided by the Delhi government were more inclusive. In particular, many informal settlement dwellers, including from Kathputli Colony, have no ration cards. In the camp, over 300 households could get free rations from government stores via a system of e-coupons devised by the Delhi government in 2020 for those without ration cards. However, the availability of sufficient stocks in these stores was often problematic, which curtailed the scheme's efficiency. Besides, supplying food grains only does not address all nutrition needs, not to mention the cost to the beneficiary of grinding them into flour. Regarding the special allowance for rickshaw drivers, although many could benefit from it, others in the camp were left out due to setbacks in the online registration process (such as incomplete application, mismatch of information, invalid driving license, application after due date, etc.).

During the lockdown, the DDA's efforts to help the families it had displaced were meager. In 2020, it distributed food rations on both resettlement sites, but the residents considered the quantities to be grossly insufficient (at most: 5 kg of wheat, 1 kg of rice, 1 kg of lentils or chickpeas, 1 liter of oil and 1 kg of sugar) given the length of the lockdown. Furthermore, they regarded it as a way to, again, control their eligibility, as they had to show their allotment documents to get the rations. Several residents refused this help to avoid bowing to administrative power. This evokes the protection with induced domination relation that may be at work in relief operations, as observed elsewhere during the pandemic (Hillenkamp, Lobo and Schwenck 2022).

Altogether, the various government relief measures to help vulnerable families confront the lingering economic crisis, though significant, were far from sufficient. Initiatives by non-state actors proved to be decisive on both resettlement sites, as shown below.

Initiatives by non-state actors at the settlement level during the first lockdown

In the transit camp, three pro-active residents, including one educated up-and-coming leader, well connected with civil society organizations, and two influential well-known artists joined to organize relief works in the wake of the lockdown. Their first motivation was to avoid a hunger crisis in the settlement. This altruistic display of humanitarianism also served their keenness to assert their leadership through their ability to help the community. They coordinated a team of about 50 young men from the camp. They started by providing immediate food support to the most vulnerable families identified by a door-to-door survey collecting details about the family composition and economic condition, and identifying, in particular, widows and women deserted by their husbands. As the number of needy families increased with the extension of the lockdown, food distribution was broadened to more families. All those in need received rations for three months, in two-three rounds, and the campaign initiators were proud that no one went hungry in the camp. An awareness campaign about COVID-19 complemented the relief works. Apart from food packets, the team supplied masks, soaps and sanitizers while promoting their usage to fight the pandemic. The exclusively masculine team asked women to help distribute sanitary pads. In addition, the same team provided help for online applications to benefit from government relief schemes. Its leader also mobilized his political contacts, including the local Member of the Legislative Assembly (MLA) to handle discrepancies in the supply of free rations at the zonal government store.

In order to fund their relief efforts, the team began collecting money from better-off camp residents on a voluntary basis. However, they soon realized that this would be insufficient to respond to the growing demand, and that they needed outside support. They then contacted potential donors – concerned people who already knew the Kathputli Colony artists, cultural organizations and various Indian NGOs engaged in humanitarian and development work. They also launched crowdfunding through social media with an electronic platform allowing contributions from abroad.[11] The senior most recognized artist-puppeteer in the team alerted the media, which publicized the camp residents' plight. Several NGOs and charitable trusts came forward with monetary or in-kind help. The team eventually collected external support from about one hundred individuals. Monetary donations allowed them to purchase various food items and other products in bulk, stock them and prepare distribution kits.

This collective endeavor was the most significant to be organized by a group of residents at the whole transit camp level. Some camp residents initiated relief efforts on a smaller scale. For instance, a local leader conducted with his followers his own door-to-door survey to distribute food rations and medicine to the needy families in some blocks, helped by an NGO that supplied the products. Further examples of solidarity include: residents who mobilized their contacts in charity organizations to collect food and distribute it in their blocks; young people who redistributed food brought from temples and Gurudwaras; a rickshaw driver who collected meals from a government community kitchen to distribute to about 200 people during three weeks; artists who performed online and purchased rations for the community with their proceeds; a Muslim shopkeeper who borrowed 15,000 rupees from his parents and distributed it to the poor of his community to purchase fruit during Ramadan. In contrast, the Residents Welfare Association (RWA) of the transit camp, controlled by the builder (and not the outcome of mandatory elections), did not take part in the relief efforts during the lockdown. Indeed, the builder was conspicuous for his negligible support to the residents.

Another strategy, observed in particular in the Narela flats, consisted of local leaders approaching politicians on behalf of the poor to get food rations and other help. Their residents complained that being on the city outskirts they were comparatively neglected by NGOs that were more supportive of the transit camp. In Narela, two rival leaders associated with different political parties and vying for the position of the RWA president played an active role. The one affiliated with the party leading the Delhi government arranged, through an MLA, the distribution of food rations and of twice-daily hot meals in the flats complex, both provided by the Delhi government. The supply of hot meals stopped after three weeks, following a misuse of food that was publicized by the media, but the local leader took over, collected money and started a community kitchen in the housing complex. His rival got the support of politicians from the party ruling at the national level and of an ancillary NGO. Basically, he arranged the same type of relief aid for the flats' residents, namely the distribution of food rations and hot meals. Yet, most recipients were oblivious to, and unconcerned by, the source of the help.

We can draw a few lessons from the various relief initiatives described above. Initiators and whistle-blowers from the community had to team up with external actors to achieve a significant impact at the settlement level. Self-organization among the inhabitants and horizontal solidarities were fundamental in reaching the maximum number of needy families. Embedded actors have a better knowledge of the communities' requirements, which they further improved (in the transit camp) with door-to-door surveys. Monetary and in-kind contributions from outside benefactors (individuals, NGOs or institutions) were equally essential in an enduring crisis that very quickly exhausted internal financial resources. In this respect, civil society's involvement proved to be decisive, especially through the connections established by some community members. Certain local leaders' political connections played a similar role in mobilizing external resources, including public resources. Better-educated residents and local leaders also played a significant role in helping the residents avail of the government relief schemes. Other studies of vulnerable groups in Indian cities highlighted the key role of such interface actors during the pandemic (Auerbach and Thachil 2021; Naik 2020). In short, the articulation of horizontal solidarity networks within the settlement and vertical networks beyond it enabled the communities to bridge over the most critical phase of the economic and food crisis.

Unscrambling communities' responses and initiatives as a litmus test for trust and solidarities

In this last section, we take the sanitary and economic crisis as a pointer to delve deeper into issues of trust among the various players involved. We distinguish between trust in state institutions at different levels and interpersonal trust. We further examine what the coping strategies described above reveal about the foundation of interpersonal reliance and solidarity networks. Finally, we question the new solidarity networks that have emerged during the crisis: can they durably transcend the prevailing dividing lines?

What trust in institutions?

As explained by Spire (2020), in modern states that draw their legitimacy from a legal rational domination (referring to the Weberian theory), "the relation of confidence is what allows the acceptance of decision taken in the name of the general interest" (ibid., 2020: 37–38 – our translation). From this perspective, the general acceptance of the first lockdown decision among the studied communities would be interpreted as a sign of confidence in the state. Indeed, most of our respondents on both sites initially considered the lockdown to be a decision in the public interest and necessary to contain the virus. Such an acceptance reflects the people's sensitivity to the fear imparted about the virus at the outset. It further indicates their faith in expert knowledge. Also, most did not anticipate that the lockdown might be extended beyond the 21-day period initially announced. The same people were very critical of the three successive lockdown extensions. Many expressed anger toward the government for "letting them down" and "ruining their life" (joining those who criticized the lockdown from the start). The lockdown extension reinforced their view that "the [central] government does not care for the poor".[12] It further fostered in them a feeling of great injustice, as they felt that the lockdown was enforced to protect the rich, at the expense of the poor's livelihoods.

This evolving appraisal of the state decisions illustrates Spire (2020)'s distinction between "symbolic confidence" and "practical trust" in institutions. Given the pandemic context and the widespread communication about the risks in various media, people expressed an *a priori* abstract confidence in the government lockdown decision. But after experiencing the devastating consequences of the lockdown in their daily life, they contrariwise expressed a lack of an *a posteriori* practical trust. Increased mistrust of the lockdown over time was also reported from other vulnerable urban dwellers in India (Bercegol et al. 2020).

Most respondents also denounced the abruptness of the lockdown announcement – at night, with a four-hour notice – which prevented them from organizing the conditions of their containment and possibly mitigating its adverse effects. They were not only referring to their own situation, but also to the migrant workers' plight, amply reported in the media, who found themselves stranded in cities with no work and no facility to return to their village. The picture of the multitude of migrants walking back home for hundreds of kilometers, their ruthless treatment by the police on the road, the belated (after over a month) arrangement of special trains to transport them, altogether this spectacle added to their own experience of the state "through a lens of violence and control", and not "through a prism of care" (Mukhopadhyay and Naik 2020). Apart from the traumatic experience of the demolition of their settlement, at the time of the sudden lockdown decision the memory of another distressing episode surfaced, that of November 8, 2016, when the government announced without prior notice the demonetization of 500 rupees and 1,000 rupees currency notes, a measure that first hit those who depended on the cash economy, especially in the informal sector (Kumar 2017; Hilger and Nordman 2020).

These past experiences, cumulated with their hardships during the prolonged lockdown, have all contributed to our respondents' practical distrust of the state, epitomized here by the current central government and its prime minister. It confirmed their dominant vision of the state as disregarding the needs of the poor, and their conclusion that in times of crisis they cannot rely on the state to effectively support them. This critical assessment includes the DDA, which is under the purview of the federal Ministry of Housing and Urban Affairs. The DDA is indeed the first interlocutor regarding the residents' present resettlement condition and future rehabilitation, their main "access point" (Giddens 1990, 83) to the central government, the catalyzer of their everyday recriminations. We observed comparatively more practical trust in the current Delhi government, considered "more poor-friendly". Most respondents acknowledged its various relief initiatives during the lockdown. The support it provided was both more inclusive and more visible, at the "frontstage" (e.g., the fair-price shops and community kitchens), whereas the central government measures were conditional, limited and involved "backstage" financial circuits.[13] In the transit camp, NGOs were the most appreciated, although residents were mostly ignorant of their identities. Their support was conspicuous, on the frontstage; it reached the residents' doorstep and was generally appraised as sizable and vital.

Fear of the virus and interpersonal mistrust

We examine here whether fear of the virus has generated interpersonal mistrust among the communities. During the lockdown in the transit camp, the residents of some blocks did not allow outsiders (namely people from other blocks and other communities) in. Similar restrictions were initially applied to outsiders in the Narela flats complex. After the lockdown was lifted, street vendors were controlled. Residents working as rickshaw drivers were viewed with suspicion because of their contact with passengers. Instances of neighbors' surveillance and suspicion were also reported in the dense habitat of the camp. In the words of a woman resident:

> When the lockdown was imposed, the situation was like this: if someone had fever and if someone did not go out of the house for 3–4 days, neighbors used to call the ambulance, saying "this particular person has corona virus".
>
> (Authors' interview, June 28, 2020)

A few residents were, accordingly, sent to a hospital for testing, and fortunately came back with negative results. Interestingly, all our respondents declared that their families had respected the COVID prevention protocol, including wearing masks in public spaces and social distancing. But they usually blamed other people, often from other communities, for not respecting those measures. The remote survey did not allow us to verify such statements. Possibly some respondents exaggerated their own compliance with the norms. However, what remains significant is the blaming game, pointing to entrenched prejudices against other communities that turned into mistrust during the pandemic. Fear of contamination from others resurfaced during the 2021 COVID-19 wave, while fear of being stigmatized in case of illness led many affected people to hide their medical condition.[14]

Interpersonal reliance and solidarity networks

The lockdown-induced economic and food crisis further raises the question of interpersonal reliance, in vertical as well as horizontal connections. The history of the Kathputli Colony redevelopment project, including politicians' false promises, has left a durable mark. Thus, no resident from the transit camp mentioned their MLA or MP (Member of Parliament) among the persons they could rely on during this crisis. Rather, the respondents complained that no politician visited the camp to help. They were seemingly unaware of the local MLA's intervention to settle problems regarding the distribution of free rations at the zonal government store. In the Narela flats, politicians solicited by community leaders did play a significant role as intermediaries to ensure the supply of food rations and meals, but many residents did not know the origin of such arrangements. In other words, on both sites, the politicians' backstage performances failed to generate noticeable practical trust among ordinary residents.

The resettlement process has marred the reputation of several traditional local leaders suspected of corruption. The old generation of leaders was especially mistrusted, being seen as selfish and corrupt, "busy filling their own stomach"[15] during the COVID crisis. We heard accusations that one leader kept part of the food rations he had collected for his family and sold the rest instead of distributing it to the community, and that another one took cuts in the monetary donations he received in the name of the Kathputli Colony people before distributing them. These various allegations, whether true or not, reveal an atmosphere of deep distrust as well as a lack of "trust in intentions" (Nooteboom 2007), with suspicion of opportunism.

To the question "who do you rely on for help during these difficult times", several respondents answered they relied first on their family and relatives, as illustrated by the coping strategies. Tellingly, some only trust themselves or God:

"I don't rely on anyone because whatever help we get from others is temporary, but what we earn from our hard work is the thing which is very important for us" (Authors' interview, July 24, 2021), explained a casual factory worker living in the Narela flats.

Although none of the respondents denied the support received from NGOs, individual benefactors or the government, they were expressing their lack of expectation from state institutions, public figures, or people facing similar problems, and considered that assistance from NGOs could not be sustainable.

Probing further signs of horizontal solidarity among the camp – or flats – residents in times of crisis highlighted significant trends. A first and commonly reported negative assessment was the lack of unity and solidarity across the settlement. This harks back to the social divisions in Kathputli Colony before its demolition, further exacerbated by the resettlement process and – according to a local leader – "the government's divide and rule policy".[16] On a finer scale, all respondents acknowledged that solidarity ran more along intra-community lines (based on caste, religion or region of origin) than along inter-community ones. Given the then prevailing shortages, most people could not give material assistance to others than relatives, namely their primary solidarity circle. And when they could do so, it was usually limited to sharing food products, and sometimes gas for cooking, with their fellow community members or their neighbors, often from the same community. As frequently expressed in varying wordings, "when you are broken, how can you help others?"[17]

Our findings on the enduring significance of traditional solidarity channels are in line with the conclusions of other studies in India on the determinants of interpersonal trust, including one conducted in the wake of the 2016 demonetization shock (Hilger and Nordman 2020), and larger surveys highlighting the role of caste (Munshi 2019). In the last section, we focus back on the collective relief initiatives organized by the residents and question the new forms of solidarity that emerged on that occasion.

New solidarities in question

Has the main 2020 collective relief initiative in the transit camp managed to transcend old and more recent dividing lines? At the operational level, the assessment is dual. Putting aside their different backgrounds, three mentors formed the crisis cell that monitored the operation: two Rajasthani artists from the same caste, and a dedicated social entrepreneur from another community and region. However, aside from four or five others, most of the 52 young volunteers belonged to the same caste: "non-artist involvement was not there" reported one team member from the majority group,[18] "because of the Rajasthani artists' superior behavior", argued another from the marginal group.[19] Thus, the inter-community divide and mistrust endured.

Some of the residents' comments on the relief operations further highlight jealousy, suspicion and mistrust. The priority given to serving the most deprived families aroused misunderstanding and criticism. Some complained their block or community was neglected and accused other communities of monopolizing outside help. Others accused the distribution team members of favoring their relatives and their own communities. Allegations of misuse of the collected funds emerged. Such accusations led to a police case filed against one campaign organizer, the non-Rajasthani, young well-educated social entrepreneur, whose profile and active role in the camp challenged the traditional leadership and triggered rivalry, and a "conspiracy", as contended by its victim.[20]

To some extent, relief works became a competition in the camp, as illustrated by a local leader who conducted his own door-to-door survey and ration distribution instead of joining the main relief operation. The reason behind his non-cooperation relates to diverging positions regarding the slum redevelopment project. This leader strongly opposed the project, whereas the organizers of the main relief campaign aligned with the pro-project group and negotiated with the DDA.

In the Narela flats, where the two main protagonists vie for the RWA president post, the organization of relief aid was clearly more competitive than cooperative. The dividing factors between these rivals and their supporters were political affiliation and community. Allegations or suspicion of food distribution favoring one's community or one's supporters were equally reported.

Our surveys showed that mistrust between the different communities was only partly transcended for the organization of aid campaigns in 2020. Moreover, the fracture between the opponents of the redevelopment project and its proponents remained significant. During the 2021 lockdown, no solidarity drive encompassing the entire settlement emerged in the transit camp. Despite some remarkable endeavors, relief distributions were less comprehensive and rather followed community-based channels and a clientelist trend, confirming the strength of traditional solidarities and the persistence of divided leadership. In some respects, the crises exacerbated rivalries as the flow of relief funds and goods generated suspicion of opportunism and distrust in intention.

Conclusion

The displaced residents of Kathputli Colony were severely impacted by the economic crisis triggered by COVID-19. For them, as for most slum dwellers in Indian cities and workers without social protection, the first risk was not the virus, but hunger, as the strict and prolonged lockdown blocked their access to livelihoods. This immediate adverse effect, followed by a sluggish economic recovery, entailed increased indebtedness, employment casualization and destitution.

The history of this settlement, its demolition and resettlement process, affected people's trust in institutions and in their fellow residents during the pandemic. The initial *a priori* confidence in expert knowledge and in the central government measures to contain the pandemic turned into a lack of practical trust, as people suffered severe hardship despite relief schemes. *De facto*, the displaced residents expect little from the state functioning system (Giddens 1990), having confronted the state apparatus through its violent arm and its callousness. Institutions that were on the frontstage at the local level during the crisis gained more trust, especially NGOs and, to a lesser extent, the Delhi government, as their support was direct, more tangible and significant.

The residents' responses to the COVID-19-induced crisis invites us to consider these resettled communities not as passive victims, but as actors, able to devise coping strategies at the household level – although within limited options – and to launch collective initiatives at the settlement level. Indeed, solidarity drives to alleviate the crisis were remarkable. They demonstrate the residents' agency and competence to efficiently organize relief works and prevent a hunger crisis. To make it possible, the residents linked their horizontal networks with vertical solidarity networks that extended beyond the resettled communities, involving NGOs, individual benefactors and/or politicians.

At the interpersonal level, family and relatives were the first solidarity circle. Beyond it, solidarity preferentially followed community-based channels.

Inter-community mistrust surfaced in relation to contamination fears, and during the relief distribution on the resettlement sites. Traditional, as well as recent, dividing lines were only partially overcome during the aid campaigns that triggered both solidarities and rivalries. This further shows that solidarity and interpersonal trust do not necessarily go hand in hand. While they do within the primary solidarity circle, this is not evident when inter-community relations are at play. Hence, the COVID-19 emergency did prompt exceptional solidarity drives transcending community divisions, but this does not mean that inter-community mistrust has disappeared.

Our study provides a few broader lessons. Faced with the major risk of a food crisis, as was the case during the COVID-19 pandemic, the coordinated relief efforts of state and non-state actors need to include the participation of embedded actors from the affected communities to deliver better results. This corroborates the findings of other studies conducted in Indian cities during the pandemic (Auerbach and Thachil 2021; Naik 2020). However, the flow of external resources and its management by community members are likely to arouse interpersonal and inter-community distrust based on suspicion of opportunism. Crises may fuel contrary forces of solidarity and mistrust, whose longer-term effects on social cohesion require follow-up research.

Notes

1 Corresponding author. This research is part of a collaboration program on subaltern urbanism in India, between IRD (the French national Research Institute for sustainable Development) and the Centre for Policy Research in Delhi. It benefitted from IRD funding. A first version of this chapter was presented at the international online workshop *Responses of local communities to Covid-19: Exploring issues of trust in the context of risks and fear*. Université Paris Cité & Nanyang Technological University, Singapore, December1–2, 2020.
2 Source: World Health Organization website: https://covid19.who.int/region/searo/country/in (accessed January 21, 2021).
3 The relief schemes relevant for our case study are presented in the third section.
4 The colony was named after the numerous puppeteers among these artists.
5 In 2021, during the second, more deadly wave, around 20 people were reportedly severely affected by the COVID-19, and one death was identified – with a caveat for under-reporting.
6 The migrant workers' plight during the lockdown and their reverse exodus were highlighted in the media, NGO reports and academic articles (for instance: Breman 2020; SWAN 2020; Yadav and Priya 2021).
7 All residents' quotes are translated from Hindi.
8 https://www.india.gov.in/spotlight/pradhan-mantri-garib-kalyan-package-pmgkp (accessed December 7, 2021).
9 This mission aims "to ensure access to financial services [...] in an affordable manner" (https://www.pmjdy.gov.in/scheme – accessed December 7, 2021).
10 This national scheme aims at subsidizing cooking gas cylinders for households under the poverty line (https://vikaspedia.in/energy/policy-support/pradhan-mantri-ujjwala-yojana – accessed December 7, 2021).
11 Support Kathputli Colony during COVID-19: https://www.ketto.org/fundraiser/support-kathputli-colony-during-covid19 (accessed February 9, 2021).

12 These views were expressed by many respondents, sometimes in harsher wording, e.g.: "The government does not care about whether the poor are living or dying" (authors' interview, woman from Narela, November 20, 2020).
13 The distinction between frontstage and backstage performances is used by Giddens (1990, 86) and Spire (2020, 49) in their discussion on trust, both referring to Goffman's (1959) concepts.
14 Authors' interview with a local leader in the transit camp, August 25, 2021.
15 Authors' interviews from the transit camp, June 9, 2020 and July 4, 2020.
16 Authors' interview from the transit camp, September 12, 2020.
17 Authors' interview from the transit camp, August 2, 2020.
18 Authors' interview, August 6, 2020.
19 Author's interview, September 8, 2020.
20 Since he could submit all accounts and bills, there was no further legal action. Authors' interview, October 8, 2020.

References

Abraham, R., A. Basole, and S. Kesar. 2021. "Tracking Employment Trajectories in the Covid-19 Pandemic: Evidence from India Panel Data". *Centre for Sustainable Employment Working Paper No. 35*. Bengaluru: Azim Premji University.

Auerbach, A.M., and T. Thachil. 2021. "How Does Covid-19 Affect Urban Slums? Evidence from Settlement Leaders in India". *World Development* 140: 1–11. DOI: 10.1016/j.worlddev.2020.105304

Azim Premji University. 2020. *COVID-19 Livelihoods Survey, Compilation of Findings*. Bengaluru: Centre for Sustainable Employment, Azim Premji University.

Breman, J. 2020. "The Pandemic in India and Its Impact on Footloose Labour". *The Indian Journal of Labour Economics* 63: 901–919. DOI: 10.1007/s41027-020-00285-8

De Bercegol, R., A. Goreau-Ponceaud, S. Gowda, and S. Raj. 2020. "Confining the Margins, Marginalizing the Confined: The Distress of Neglected Lockdown Victims in Indian Cities". *EchoGéo [Online]*. DOI: 10.4000/echogeo.19357

De Groot, J., and C. Lemanski. 2021. "COVID-19 Responses: Infrastructure Inequality and Privileged Capacity to Transform Everyday Life in South Africa". *Environment & Urbanization* 33(1): 255–272. DOI: 10.1177/0956247820970094

Downs-Tepper, H., A. Krishna, and E. Rains. 2022. "A Threat to Life and Livelihoods: Examining the Effects of the First Wave of COVID-19 on Health and Wellbeing in Bengaluru and Patna Slums". *Environment & Urbanization*. 34(1): 190–208. DOI: 10.1177/09562478211048778

Dupont, V., and S Gowda. 2020. "Slum-free City Planning Versus Durable Slums. Insights from Delhi". *International Journal of Sustainable Urban Development* 12(1): 34–51. DOI: 10.1080/19463138.2019.1666850

Dupont, V., and S. Gowda. 2021. "Slum Redevelopment and Differentiated Resettlement in Delhi. The Case of Kathputli Colony Rehabilitation Project". In *Urban Resettlement in the Global South*, edited by R. Beier, A. Spire, and M. Bridonneau, 25–45. Abingdon: Routledge.

Dupont, V., S. Banda, Y. Vaidya, and S. Gowda. 2014. "Unpacking Participation in Kathputli Colony. Delhi's First Slum Redevelopment Project, Act I". *Economic and Political Weekly* 49(24): 39–47.

Duque Franco, I., C. Ortiz, J. Samper, and G. Millan. 2020. "Mapping Repertoires of Collective Action Facing the COVID-19 Pandemic in Informal Settlements in Latin American Cities". *Environment & Urbanization* 32(2): 523–546. DOI: 10.1177/0956247820944823

Economic Times. 2020a. "PM Modi's Seven-point Plan to Win the Covid-19 Battle". *The Economic Times*, 14 April. https://economictimes.indiatimes.com/news/politics-and-nation/pm-modis-seven-point-plan-to-win-the-covid-19-battle/articleshow/75137621.cms

Economic Times. 2020b "Elderly, Differently-abled, Widows to Get 3 Months' Pension in Advance". *The Economic Times*, 27 March. https://economictimes.indiatimes.com/wealth/personal-finance-news/elderly-differently-abled-widows-to-get-3-months-pension-in-advance/articleshow/74847650.cms?from=mdr

Giddens, A. 1990. *The Consequences of Modernity*. Cambridge: Polity Press.

Goffman, E. 1959. *The Presentation of Self in Everyday Life*. New York: Doubleday Anchor.

Guérin, I., S. Michiels, A. Natal, C.J. Nordman, and G. Venkatasubramanian. 2020. "Surviving Debt, Survival Debt in Times of Lockdown". *CEB Working Paper No. 20-009*. Brussels: Centre Emile Bernheim & Université Libre de Bruxelles.

Hebbar, N. 2020. "Coronavirus: PM's Address to the Nation Updates: Lockdown Extended to Entire Country for Next 21 Days, Says Modi". *The Hindu*, 24 March. https://www.thehindu.com/news/national/prime-minister-narendra-modi-live-updates-march-24-2020/article31153585.ece#!

Hilger, A., and C.J. Nordman. 2020. "The Determinants of Trust: Evidence from Rural South India". *IZA Discussion Paper No. 13150*. Bonn: IZA Institute of Labour Economics.

Hillenkamp, I., B. Schwenck, and N. Lobo,. 2022. "COVID-19 Responses of Women Solidarity Networks in Brazil. Levels of Protection and (Mis)trust in a Polarized Society". In *COVID-19 Responses of Local Communities around the World. Exploring Trust in the Context of Risks and Fear*, edited by G. Guiheux, K.E. Kuah, and F. Lim, 99–119. New York and Abington: Routledge.

HLRN. 2020. *India's COVID-19 Lockdown: Human Rights Assessment and Compilation of State Relief Measures*. New Delhi: Housing and Land Right Network.

Kesar, S., R. Abraham, R. Lahoti, P. Nath, and A. Basole. 2020. "Pandemic, Informality, and Vulnerability: Impact of COVID-19 on Livelihoods in India". *Centre for Sustainable Employment Working Paper No. 27*. Bengaluru: Azim Premji University.

Khera, R., and A. Somanchi. 2020. "Covid-19 and Aadhaar: Why the Union Government Relief Package Is an Exclusionary Endeavour". *Economic and Political Weekly* 55(17) [on line] https://www.epw.in/engage/article/covid-19-and-aadhaar-why-union-governments-relief

Kumar, A. 2017. "Economic Consequences of Demonetisation: Money Supply and Economic Structure". *Economic & Political Weekly* 52(1): 14–17.

Luhmann, N. 1979. *Trust and Power*. Chichester: Wiley.

Mander, H. 2020. "State's Measures to Fight Corona Are Stripping the Poor of Dignity". *The Indian Express*, March 27. https://indianexpress.com/article/opinion/columns/coronavirus-covid-19-lockdown-poor-6333452/

Mukhopadhya, P., and M. Naik. 2020. "Migrant Workers Distrust a State that Does not Take Them into Account". *The Indian Express*, March 31. https://indianexpress.com/article/opinion/columns/coronavirus-lockdown-covid-19-deaths-cases-mass-exodus-migrant-workers-6339152/

Munshi, K. 2019. "Caste and the Indian Economy". *Journal of Economic Literature* 57(4): 781–834. DOI: 10.1257/jel.20171307

Naik, M. 2020. "State–society Interactions and Bordering Practices in Gurugram's Pandemic Response". *Urbanisation* 5(2): 181–190. DOI: doi.org/10.1177/2455747120974531

Ngullie, O.G., and A.A. Ansari. 2021. "Impact of the Pandemic on Livelihood and Food Security: An Empirical Analysis of the PDS in Delhi". *Indian Journal of Public Administration* 67(3): 314–323. DOI: 10.1177/00195561211045797

Nooteboom, B. 2007. "Social Capital, Institutions and Trust". *Review of Social Economy* 65(1): 29–53. DOI: 10.1080/00346760601132154

Spire, A. 2020. "La confiance dans l'État : une relation pratique et symbolique". In *Crises de confiance ?*, edited by C. Senik, 37–55. Paris: La Découverte.

SWAN. 2020. *21 Days and Counting: COVID-19 Lockdown, Migrant Workers, and the Inadequacy of Welfare Measures in India*. Stranded Workers Action Network. http://strandedworkers.in/mdocuments-library/

Unni, J. 2020. "Impact of Lockdown Relief Measures on Informal Enterprises and Workers". *Economic and Political Weekly*, 55(51) [On line] URL: https://www.epw.in/engage/article/impact-lockdown-relief-measures-informal-enterprises-workers

Wilkinson, A., and contributors. 2020. "Local Response in Health Emergencies: Key Considerations for Addressing the COVID-19 Pandemic in Informal Urban Settlements". *Environment & Urbanization* 32(2): 503–522. DOI: 10.1177/0956247820922843

Wratten, E. 1995. "Conceptualizing Urban Poverty". *Environment and Urbanization* 7(1): 11–38. DOI: 10.1177/095624789500700118

Yadav, S., and K.R. Priya. 2021. "Migrant Workers and COVID-19: Listening to the Unheard Voices of Invisible India". *Journal of the Anthropological Survey of India* 70(1): 62–71. DOI: 10.1177/2277436X20968984

6 COVID-19 responses of women's solidarity networks in Brazil

Levels of protection and (mis)trust in a polarized society

Isabelle Hillenkamp[1], *Beatriz Schwenck and Natália Lobo*

Introduction: trust, protection and solidarity – research question and argument

The COVID-19 pandemic has been putting the social relations of protection to the test worldwide, not only by increasing the risk to and vulnerability of populations in the health field, but also in the social and economic spheres more broadly. The pandemic has highlighted contrasting responses from states, local communities and civil society organizations, and varying degrees of effectiveness, solidarity and concerted or violent actions. In this chapter, we consider that the institutions upon which social relations of protection have been built (the social state, different types of families, communities and civil society organizations) are grounded in diverse levels and forms of trust. The way in which these relations have evolved in recent months in the face of the COVID-19 pandemic has been conditioned by how those institutions have been constructed over the long term.

In Brazil, the social relations of trust, protection and solidarity stem from the colonial history of slavery and patriarchy combined (Franco 1997; Saffioti 2004). This long history has also determined unequal access to social rights on the basis of state presence in the territories, in close association with ethnic-racial, class and gender discrimination. Such discrimination has been challenged with the democratization of Brazil, in the aftermath of the military dictatorship (1964–1985). From the 1980s, so-called "autonomous", women-only social movements emerged, denouncing the gender bias of the state and of class-based social movements, which were not representing the women's interests (Jalil 2013). They campaigned firstly for women's access to social rights, and then, progressively, for the recognition of a more inclusive, non-capitalist model of economic organization. Starting in the late 1990s, and then under the 2003 to 2016 Workers' Party governments, mixed movements of women and men joined forces under the banners of the "solidarity economy" and "agroecology". They stood for anti-capitalist values based on self-management and cooperation (the solidarity economy) and on a sustainable mode of food production, respecting the ecosystem regeneration cycles (agroecology) (Hillenkamp and Nobre 2021). Women's movements

DOI: 10.4324/9781003291220-6

stressed the importance of democratizing all relations of domination within the solidarity economy and agroecology: not only capitalist, but also patriarchal and racial (Hillenkamp and Nobre 2021). Thanks to their alliances with NGOs and higher education institutions, and to local and federal public policies that stemmed largely from the Workers' Party from 2003 to 2016, these movements have branched out into a number of territories (França Filho et al. 2006). At a national level, a rural women's union meeting known as Marcha das Margaridas, has been held in Brasilia every four or five years since 2000, with up to 100,000 women participants (Butto Zarzar 2017).

With the COVID-19 pandemic, this historical intersection of state-building and the development of social movements has signified a complex interplay between the modern project for a universal social state and highly diverse territorial relations within local communities and solidarity networks. We offer, here, a case study of the forms of trust, protection and solidarity that two local Brazilian women's solidarity networks have mobilized. They are AMESOL, the Association of Women in Solidarity Economy of São Paulo, an urban solidarity economy network, and RAMA, the Agroecological Network of Women Farmers, a local rural agroecology network, which have both faced up to the increased risk and insecurity brought about by the COVID-19 pandemic. We argue that a certain type of trust is specific to AMESOL and RAMA. It stems from women backing a political discourse that is critical of domination along gender, class and race lines (political trust), and gradually implementing the solidarity economy and agroecology proposals which are contained in this discourse (pragmatic trust). Moreover, uncertainty over access to state social protection under President Bolsonaro has inflamed distrust among some of the population, boosting the meaningfulness of alternative forms of trust in solidarity networks and local communities.

This chapter is structured as follows: after this introduction, the second section sets out our theoretical approach, while the third section presents AMESOL and RAMA, reflecting on the conditions of our survey and its methodology. The fourth section analyzes how trust came to be built within AMESOL and RAMA prior to the COVID-19 pandemic. The fifth section considers how the pandemic has affected RAMA and AMESOL and how trust, protection and solidarity have been renewed. The sixth section shifts the focus of our analysis to the local communities where AMESOL and RAMA women live. It highlights the state's willful ignorance of local demands for protection, and the very different type of trust that exists in these communities. The seventh section explains the links between those forms of trust, protection and solidarity observed at the local level, and trust and mistrust in the Brazilian State protection system and governments. In the eighth section we offer our concluding remarks, including our key argument and the lessons learned from our research.

Theoretical approach

Our theoretical approach takes its starting point in Anthony Giddens's (1990) analysis of different forms of trust. Beginning with an understanding of trust as a social relationship that reduces "ontological insecurity", which is inherent to human life, Giddens situates his analysis in the context of modernity. For Giddens, modernity is "a double-edged phenomenon", featuring a dialectical movement of "disembedding and reembedding of social relations from local conditions of time and place" (Giddens 1990, 10). Within this framework, Giddens's analysis of trust distinguishes between *facework commitments* ("trust relations which are sustained by or expressed in social connections established in circumstances of copresence") and *faceless commitments* ("the development of faith in symbolic tokens or expert systems, which, taken together, I shall call abstract systems"; Giddens 1990, 10). Giddens stresses the movement of disembedding and reembedding of social relations of trust in local conditions of time and place, and the interplay between faceless and facework commitments:

> all disembedding mechanisms interact with reembedded contexts of action, which may act either to support or to undermine them; [...] faceless commitments are similarly linked in an ambiguous way with those demanding facework.
>
> (Giddens 1990, 80)

Giddens also assumes that there is a discontinuity between forms of risk and trust in "pre-modern cultures" and "modern cultures". In pre-modern cultures, risks would have been caused by natural dangers, human violence and "risk of a fall from religious grace", while in modern cultures, risks are associated with "the reflexivity of modernity", human violence and personal meaningless. While in pre-modern cultures, trust has been based on kinship relations, local communities, religious cosmologies and tradition, in modern cultures, trust would be grounded in "personal relations of friendships and sexual intimacy", abstract systems and "future-oriented thought" (Giddens 1990, 102). Giddens particularly stresses the importance of trust in abstract systems in modern cultures:

> It will be a basic part of my argument that the nature of modern institutions is deeply bound up with the mechanisms of trust in abstract systems, especially trust in expert systems.
>
> (Giddens 1990, 83)

Following Giddens, we will define trust as a social relationship that reduces ontological insecurity. We pay attention to the movement of disembedding and reembedding of social relations of trust and we approach trust both in terms of abstract systems and personal relationships. But we do not limit personal relationships of trust to friendship or sexual intimacy as Giddens does, or as a means of stabilizing social ties in modern cultures. We challenge the sharp distinction he makes between pre-modern and modern cultures, and call attention to the permanence of a diversity of trust relationships embedded in personal relationships in contemporary Brazil. We call for a broader, more critical understanding of how trust, risk and protection are embedded in a diversity of social relations in local communities, and how solidarity-based organizations interact with the dynamic of trust and mistrust, and of inclusion and exclusion from modern state-led social protection system. Our shift away from Giddens's framework is as such directly linked to our focus on inequalities, from the global to the local level. While part of the world's population is integrated into market globalization, with increasing or often almost exclusive recourse to the disembedded public and private protection schemes that Giddens discusses, another, subaltern part is excluded from such institutions, or receives only inadequate risk coverage. This part of the population draws instead, or simultaneously, on other, personal, relationships of trust and protection, which may be solidarity-based or embedded in high inequality.

Our theoretical approach is informed by feminist and decolonial criticism of inequalities based in racial, class and gender discriminations. The Modernity-Coloniality school of thought criticized Giddens's assumption of discontinuity between modern and pre-modern cultures for its lack of attention to inequalities and its questionable claim to universality (Escobar 2003). Feminist and decolonial theories have highlighted the invisible work of care taken on by subaltern women as they contend with the vulnerability of life and rebuild trust and protection relationships on a day-to-day basis. They have highlighted the importance of care work, which is steered by a subtle mix of reciprocity, altruism and obligation, in dealing with the concrete risks and insecurity of everyday life (Fisher and Tronto 1990; Lugones 2007; Federici 2012).

Subaltern studies have used the concept of subalternity to highlight the mechanism of invisibility and repression of the activities and voices of subordinate groups, whose history has taken place on the margins of dominant institutions and narratives (Spivak, 1988). Nancy Fraser's discussion of the public sphere went on to define subalternity as a political expression of subordination. She coined the concept of "subaltern counterpublics" as "discursive arenas where members of subordinated social groups invent and circulate counterdiscourses, which in turn permit them to formulate oppositional interpretations of their identities, interests, and needs" (Fraser 1990, 67).

Luciane Lucas dos Santos, a Brazilian feminist postcolonial economist, connected the political and socioeconomic dimensions of subalternity, addressing "other productivities, temporalities and knowledge, as well as different logics of production, consumption, and circulation of goods" (Lucas dos Santos 2018, 5). From this viewpoint, the subordinated social groups' capacity to form subaltern counterpublics is inextricably linked to "fostering solidarity and popular economic initiatives to face their social and economic vulnerability" (Lucas dos Santos 2018, 5).

Case study and methodology

AMESOL and RAMA, the focuses of our case study, are two local solidarity networks of subaltern women in Southeast Brazil. AMESOL, the Association of Women in Solidarity Economy of São Paulo, has around 50 women members, mostly craftswomen and cooks who live on the outskirts of the São Paulo megalopolis. RAMA, the Agroecological Network of Women Farmers, has some 70 women farmer members from rural communities in Barra do Turvo, a municipality of Vale do Ribeira, an Atlantic Forest territory in the State of São Paulo. Both have connections to Sempreviva Organisação Feminista (SOF), a Brazilian feminine (women only) and feminist NGO that runs projects in support of women solidarity networks at the same time as contributing to the development of the feminist movement. SOF actively participates in the World March of Women, a transnational feminist network that broadly defines itself as anti-patriarchal, anti-capitalist and anti-racist (Masson and Conway 2017). SOF encourages AMESOL and RAMA members to become involved in feminist, solidarity economy and agroecological movements as subaltern counterpublics and to claim their economic and political autonomy as working-class, often racialized women.

On the empirical level, this text draws mainly on a remote survey carried out with AMESOL and RAMA between March and November 2020. In addition, data from earlier projects (Schwenck 2019; Hillenkamp and Lobo 2019; Hillenkamp and Nobre 2021) are used to account for the construction of trust in AMESOL and RAMA before the COVID-19 pandemic. Testimonies recorded in March 2021 from RAMA women during the filming of a presentation of the survey's results,[2] are also quoted. The survey consisted of individual recorded interviews held on WhatsApp or by telephone with 43 AMESOL and 33 RAMA members; participant observation of their (once or twice monthly) online meetings; follow-up of their WhatsApp groups, and the "Responsible Consumption Groups" in São Paulo who buy products from RAMA. Finally, telephone interviews were conducted with three key informants in the health and education sectors in Barra do Turvo, where RAMA is based.

This survey was possible thanks to our integration within these networks and organizations over several years in the framework of action-research projects. Action-research denotes a method of producing knowledge that, beyond contributing to academic debate, is oriented toward social transformation: in our case, the economic and political autonomy of subaltern women through the solidarity economy and agroecology. Such research feeds into action through the type of questions asked, by relating to some of the concerns of social actors, and by reporting the research findings and debating them at different levels (Mies 1991; Fals Borda 1999). In this remote survey, the restitution of results began with podcasts and videos posted by us in RAMA and AMESOL WhatsApp groups, as a way to provoke debates, as well as virtual meetings with SOF and other actors from local social movements. Given the context of increased vulnerability due to the pandemic, we also responded to some immediate requests raised by the women, in particular for information and support in accessing the government's emergency aid and for information on the reasons for the interruption of medical services in some communities and on prospects for recovery (see later in this chapter). The reliability of our remotely gathered data is grounded in the relationships of trust that we built up with AMESOL and RAMA members over these processes.

Trust-building in AMESOL and RAMA before the pandemic: political and pragmatic dimensions

AMESOL and RAMA were created in 2013 and 2015, respectively. Both were predicated on the interactions between SOF staff and women local leaders, with the goal of strengthening a "feminist solidarity economy". This model brings together solidarity economic practices based on cooperation and self-management with championing a fair sexual division of labor and placing a value on the domestic and care work of subaltern women. RAMA carries out agricultural production, taking a feminist solidarity economic model combined with agroecology for sustainable food production. The feminist solidarity economy model supported by SOF has been discussed in Brazil since the 1990s, particularly within the framework of the Feminist Economy Network (REF, *Rede de Economia Feminista*). It as such adheres to a radical vision to transform the dominant socioeconomic order, and gender, race and class as power relations.

AMESOL's members are urban entrepreneurs (craftswomen, cooks, seamstresses). They have been involved in the solidarity economy in local organizations or networks or benefited from public policies to support the solidarity economy under the Workers' Party governments. Moreover, some have campaigned in feminist organizations, notably the World March of Women. In Vale do Ribeira, RAMA members belong to traditional so-called *quilombola* communities (recognized as descendants of black slaves), to local agroforestry organizations, but also to informal handicrafts, cooking and mutual aid groups. These women have a shared experience of subalternity, typified by submission to men in their families and communities and to employers or landowners, a lack of income or control over their incomes, and often overwork and domestic violence. This experience differs from that of SOF female workers, who occupy a higher social position and generally have greater economic and personal autonomy. Many AMESOL and RAMA women did not initially consider themselves feminists.

> Our agenda is how to insert women, particularly *quilombola* women, who have another reality, in the feminist movement [...] We are still learning, this agenda is very new.
>
> (*Quilombola* leader Nayara,[3] November 2018)

For these women, the feminist solidarity economy first and foremost constitutes a change in practice. For example, RAMA informants Maria and Ivonete emphasized the importance of "having an income" and "being able to travel" (in order to participate in training, meetings, sales or marches), and RAMA informants Margarida and Dandara highlighted the fact of "being able to share housework with one's partners" and "not accepting violence" (various RAMA interviews, 2018–2020).

Trust between SOF staff and AMESOL and RAMA women is founded on the shared feminist solidarity economy project, but both parties have interpreted that project differently in terms of their experiences and social positions. Within this configuration, trust has been inextricably *political*, i.e., based on a shared vision of the transformation of economic and social relations, and *pragmatic*, i.e., subject to the gradual implementation of this transformation. SOF has committed to helping the women take action (local groups, networks), to offering training in production (agroecology, handicrafts, etc.), self-management (sales organization, collective work) and marketing their products (feminist and solidarity economy fairs, Responsible Consumption Groups networks). It has fostered trust by demonstrating the NGO's sincerity and its ability to put its proposals into practice. Trust was thus built on a *rapprochement* between a radical social transformation proposal, and its progressive implementation on the basis of local possibilities for action. This trust was based on personal relationships in each women's network, between the women and the SOF staff, and on the concrete actions (training, fairs, meetings, etc.) that made it possible to put the political proposal into practice.

This pragmatic trust-building, founded on progressive social transformation and personal relations, is made manifest in how these organizations include their new members. Newcomers to AMESOL are asked if they are willing to participate in meetings, working committees and contribute to the association's collective fund. The willingness to accept immediate involvement in the collective self-managed work and running of the organization is the key criteria and basis for trust. On a second level, knowledge of and interest in the feminist solidarity economy as a model for social transformation is presented, as an open question and an aspiration to be achieved over time. RAMA generally recruits new members by inviting them from within a framework of close relationships (neighbors, relatives) at the community level. The woman who offers the invitation introduces the newcomer to the organization and explains how the local group and the network work. She usually stresses that "it's not just about selling", but about "working together" and "fighting violence against women". Such direct transmission is a clear instance of facework commitment. It is reinforced by RAMA's written rules, which require new membership to be collective (a group of at least three people) and that new members take part in collective work and meetings for six months before starting to market their products.

Moreover, SOF's work with AMESOL and RAMA has been based on alliances with activist organizations and networks such as the World March of Women, the network of around ten Responsible Consumption Groups in São Paulo megalopolis, and civil society supporting organizations in the field of solidarity economics and agroecology. These organizations have been purchasing AMESOL and RAMA products, providing technical support, marketing opportunities and/or opening up spaces for them to participate in political campaigning. They are typical of what Brazilian sociologist Ilse Scherer-Warren (2008) has called networks of social movements, where civil society organizes on the basis of shared interests and values and of different levels of belonging and institutionalization. Such networks bring together action at the local/community level with broader mobilization. The relationship within these broader networks is based on the same type of political and pragmatic trust. It depends on the personal relationships between AMESOL and RAMA women and activists within these social movements, but also on the intermediation of key people, who are usually NGO activists and staff. Before the pandemic, these networks already used remote communication platforms for meetings (WhatsApp groups, videoconferencing) and for sales operations (Facebook). But they also made efforts to hold face-to-face meetings, including the annual Responsible Consumption Groups of São Paulo visit, where consumers would spend three days alongside the RAMA women farmers in their homes and communities. This type of encounter used to be both operational (deciding on production, sales, prices, etc.) and emotionally meaningful (singing, listening to music, reading poems, dancing, making physical contact, sometimes praying together). They highlighted that mutual knowledge, experiences of local contexts and dialogue are essential elements of mutual understanding, trust and collective action.

Renewing trust, solidarity and protection in AMESOL and RAMA during the COVID-19 pandemic

From March 2020, the COVID-19 pandemic brutally affected the living conditions of AMESOL and RAMA's women and their families. Sales and incomes dropped, especially at AMESOL; other jobs and income-generating activities were lost. Schools were closed, doctors' visits were interrupted and health posts were temporarily closed. Home-based care work increased sharply due to school closures, the disorganization of the healthcare system and the care needed for people suffering from COVID-19 and other illnesses, as well as because of the rise in people being at home all day. In our interviews, RAMA and AMESOL women have typically responded that they were the ones, with the help of their daughters or other women in their families, who took on this extra workload. The children's school lessons were a particular burden for many mothers, who had themselves dropped out of school early.

> The school lesson … in this case at lunchtime I would sit down to have lunch, to rest, and I would say [to my children], "Get the lesson and I will help you". We also don't have much study, I found it very complicated.
>
> (RAMA member Dandara, mother of seven children, March 2021)

At the same time, local forms of mutual aid were restricted by the risks of contagion from the virus. This led some women and their families, especially in São Paulo, to isolate themselves completely. Others, notably in *quilombola* communities in rural areas, faced the dilemma of either maintaining contact with their relatives in neighboring homes at the risk of infecting them, or breaking off contact, jeopardizing the basis of the community economy. Overall, the pandemic undermined close, family-based and community-based trust relationships, increased insecurity and women's workloads, while generating existential uncertainty about the future. Many women stressed their physical, but also psychological fatigue in terms of stress, anxiety and even depression.

> Ah, it's a little hard because we used to participate in meetings, in masses … everything stopped. We can't see each other at all, it's very complicated. I also had the COVID, here, it is very difficult.
>
> (RAMA member Zilda, March 2021)

Due to the pandemic, AMESOL, RAMA, SOF and all their political allies had to implement social distancing. All collective work and trainings were interrupted, sales were halted and reorganized and all operational meetings had to migrate onto virtual spaces. AMESOL switched to video calls for its meetings. To do so, the women sourced mobile phones for members without ones. They also used the association's collective fund, derived from 5% of their sales, to purchase refill internet data packages for those unable to afford them. Some women with digital skills set up tutorials on using applications and social networks. A seamstress, who is a member of AMESOL, stated:

> the women of AMESOL helped me to use these [social] networks, which for me were a burden. You made it look so easy [referring to other members of the association]. Your teaching made me see that it wasn't a headache, teaching me how to photograph, how to post, which resources to use, about Instagram […] Thank you so much. I thank you all for working together.
>
> (AMESOL member Cintia, WhatsApp message, 2021)

For RAMA, scarce internet coverage in the rural area forced the women to set up an original online meeting format, where they exchanged WhatsApp audio messages at an agreed time and followed a pre-arranged agenda. Some women would gather in small groups in the home of a woman with an internet connection, while others would walk to a roadside or the top of a hill to get a signal. SOF, in partnership with a Brazilian feminist hacker collective called "Vedetas" also set up a community network project, which allowed for the installation of three internet distribution points for collective use in a *quilombola* community in Barra do Turvo.

Solidarity and the use of virtual communication made it possible to develop two main types of responses to the pandemic. The first type of response focused on *ensuring the continuity of production and sales*. RAMA sold a wide range of products (nearly 300) as a way to enhance the value of women's typical, diversified food production. Selling a wide variety of products in relatively small quantities involves complex logistics. WhatsApp communications have allowed RAMA women to agree internally on newly defined simplified food baskets, on how to load them while respecting social distance and on new collection routes to avoid the movement of women from high-risk COVID-19 groups (notably elderly, diabetic and obese women). Logistical and financial support from the SOF was essential to help coordinate these actions between places over 300 kilometers apart and to deal with unforeseen events, including the withdrawal of the municipality truck that was used for deliveries. As a result of this, and thanks to the Responsible

Consumption Groups' interest and commitment in buying products from women with a wide range of products, in some months, their sales volume was over three times higher than in a pre-pandemic month.

AMESOL, which as a network was mainly geared toward handicrafts, shifted some of its production to manufacturing masks. Collective work was reorganized based on a sequential division of labor (cutting, sewing, sanitizing, packaging) to meet large orders, while enabling the women to work from home, using SOF's office as a physical hub for the logistics of collective production. This addressed the need for social isolation and helped the women cope with increased levels of care work at home. SOF also supported AMESOL by introducing the women to larger production chains, signing up for public mask procurement and building production and product marketing partnerships.

A second type of response to the pandemic involved *mutual aid and donations for vulnerable individuals and families*. The SOF in São Paulo, with backing from AMESOL and the World March of Women, launched an online fundraising campaign to help AMESOL women cope with the drop in their incomes. The campaign was publicized online through the social movement network. The money raised was distributed equally among AMESOL members (R$300 per woman, equivalent to around €50). Funds from an international cooperation project were also used to purchase RAMA products, which were donated in the form of food baskets to AMESOL members. These baskets came together with a leaflet asserting the political, solidarity-based and feminist scopes of this campaign, setting it apart from charity actions. Some extra purchases made from RAMA by the Responsible Consumption Groups were also donated to others in need (street people, members of the housing movement, refugees, inhabitants of indigenous villages).

Overall, these actions renewed the women's trust in their organization, in SOF and in the network of social movements. RAMA's increased sales and production have proven the effectiveness of these actions, in contrast to the uncertainty surrounding federal government policy:

> At the same time that we feel sad because of this situation, we feel strong because if we say "hello" to RAMA, wow! We hear a lot of information, we hear a lot of words that comfort us.
>
> (RAMA member Ivonete, March 2021)

> They [the federal government] cut the emergency aid, but ours here is continuing, helping the same thing and it's … going even better, because people liked the products better and there were more requests for us to sell.
>
> (RAMA member Vitória, March 2021)

Trust in AMESOL also held steady despite sales dropping, as the products they offered were less essential than those of RAMA, and due to the pandemic's strong health impact on São Paulo's megalopolis. Their demonstrated commitment to the solidarity and feminist economy during this critical period, by their efforts to reorganize production, sales and solidarity campaigns, counted the most.

> As a person, thank God I feel empowered, together with the women of AMESOL, with the women of the feminist social movement. I have never distrusted them. I have been part of this movement for many years and each time I get stronger, more and more I believe that we never walk alone. I am very happy to be part of this social movement, especially the solidarity economy network. We are being reborn, reformulating ourselves. Just like this moment of the masks, when many people were looking for people to make them, and those people were us. We, women, who are in the front line to be able to produce and give a welfare to society. [...] We are present here holding each other's hands and saying "don't give up, together we will walk".
>
> (AMESOL member Daiane, August 2020)

While digital communication allowed the women to pursue collective action despite social distancing, limitations also surfaced. The need to focus on operational functions such as sales, production and income, due to the economic emergency and the impossibility of holding face-to-face meetings, led to some neglect of political capacity-building. Trust was renewed on the pragmatic basis of operational actions and results, rather than social transformation. This imbalance can, for instance, be felt in terms of the women who joined RAMA during the pandemic, who tend to see the network mainly as a space for selling.

Using digital communication to nurture political allies for the social movement network was often the job of SOF staff, who took on a *de facto* mediating position between these allies and the women of AMESOL and RAMA. Direct contact also took place and was encouraged by the NGO but was limited by difficulties in communication and in building new personal relationships without face-to-face contact.

Moreover, despite collective efforts to widen online access and to encourage the mastery of new technologies, the lack of access in some urban and rural territories, the cost of adequate equipment and data packages and the lack of knowledge about these technologies could not always be overcome. Some women remained excluded from the digital communication, and even for women who had access and remained in regular contact with their organization, mutual understanding and connection was impeded by the lack of face-to-face contact. The risk of exhausting relationships of trust became obvious, especially when controversial issues arose (e.g., discussions on political parties, religion or racial differences in AMESOL), or when conflicts needed to be mediated (e.g., to ensure that participation in collective work was equitably distributed in RAMA). SOF workers had to intervene in individual and group conversations with AMESOL and RAMA women to address such conflicts. These would have previously been easily dealt with during the face-to-face meetings where they erupted.

Trust and protection in "local communities": different types of relationships and answers to invisible demands

While participating in solidarity networks, RAMA and AMESOL women continue to live in territories and "local communities" where the reconfiguration of social relations of protection and (mis)trust in the context of the pandemic has been forging daily interactions. The difficulty of naming these "local communities" out of a diversity of self-designations (*comunidade*, *quebrada*, *favela*, *bairro*, *vila*, *quilombo*) is illustrative of the many meanings and categories this discussion involves. This wide-ranging debate, which we will not enter into here, is a reminder of the long-standing socio-territorial inequality in Brazil. This has brought about diverse needs and responses (or lack thereof) to the COVID-19 crisis, resulting in different pandemic experiences between these communities and in relation with other, better-off neighborhoods. Beyond this diversity, the common characteristic of the communities where RAMA and AMESOL women live lies in their position of subalternity in relation to the Brazilian State, which ignores their voices and rights.

Vale do Ribeira, where RAMA is based, has large farms (*fazendas*) and companies in the mining and agro-industrial sectors alongside poor communities in so-called rural districts (*bairros rurais*) and *quilombola* communities. The recognition as *quilombola* communities was achieved through the work of the Brazilian black movement from the 1970s onwards, and was enshrined in the 1988 Brazilian Constitution, which granted a collective right to land ownership. Nevertheless, this political identity and the associated rights are constantly under dispute: the pride of resistance versus stigma and denial of rights (da Silva 2019). Such denial has considerably increased under the government of President Bolsonaro, who has questioned the existence of structural racism in Brazil and has widely suspended the recognition of *quilombola* lands (de Oliveira, Barboza & Alentejano 2020). The rural districts, on the other hand, have mainly been shaped by migrant farmers and their heirs from other regions of the country. These spaces are permeated by agrarian conflicts, and unconsolidated land and social rights, which expose them to *de facto* eviction by the state or by the large farms or companies in the region. In addition, poor communities in Vale do Ribeira, which is largely situated in forest protection areas, are submitted to repression from the environmental police (Bernini 2015).

The diverse outskirts of São Paulo megalopolis where AMESOL women live, in Brazil's biggest metropolitan region with a population around 21 million, are all home to migrant populations from other regions of the country. They have little or no urban infrastructure, and limited access to public services (Caldeira 2000). The issue is worsened by the high cost of mobility (high ticket fares, long distances, non-existent or precarious public transport). Violence, which is imposed through police repression and at the same time regulated by the "world of crime" itself (Feltran 2010), further constrains the political expression of the inhabitants.

Such situations are illustrative of a shared position of social marginality in relation to other, sometimes neighboring, territories and of subalternity as a lack of relevance in the eyes of the state and local governments: lives which do not matter. The pandemic has worsened this lack of recognition and the situation of vulnerable groups – such as women, black people, young people and informal market laborers – in these communities. On a national level, women's unemployment and inactivity rate in 2020 reached 60% (Costa, Barbosa and Hecksher 2021). Data gathered in April and May 2020 by the SOF and the media organization *Gênero e Número* in an online survey with over 2,000 women highlighted the particular difficulties black and rural women have faced. 40% of the women declared that the pandemic has endangered their subsistence, 55% among black women. In concrete terms, in rural areas the main difficulty has been paying basic bills (electricity, gas), while in the urban areas, the main issue has been paying the rent. Moreover, women's care work has significantly increased. Fifty percent of all women and 62% of women living in rural areas have started to take care of someone during the pandemic (Gênero e Número and SOF 2020).

On the micro-sociological level, RAMA and AMESOL women's testimonials point to a dramatic lack of access to the public health system (health posts closed, interruption of doctors' visits) and difficulty ensuring social distancing, particularly in São Paulo, where some families' homes cannot support everyone at once. For example, one of the AMESOL women lives with her family of 11 in a 40-square-meter two-room flat. In these urban territories too, many people have not stopped working during the pandemic and have been taking crowded public transport. We also observed cases of cash shortages and hunger, whereas in Vale do Ribeira family farming provides some degree of food autonomy.

The increased level of needs unmet by the state in poor urban and rural territories has sparked a series of local community responses, to try to fill this gap by mobilizing very different types of mostly personal relations of trust. In the outskirts of São Paulo, invisible but crucial demands for items such as soap and food have been partly met by local self-organization, e.g., neighborhood associations which collected and donated cleaning and hygiene kits. Here, solidarity has been horizontal, both requiring and fostering interpersonal trust. But these actions have had limited reach and scope. More vertical types of action also exist in local communities. These include church donations of food baskets, whereby protection and trust intertwine with reproducing social hierarchies. Finally, drug networks have long functioned as a social integration mechanism in the poor outskirts of Brazilian big cities (Zaluar 2004). In the name of "brotherhood"[4] these networks offer help to people in need in the community, at the same time combining relations of protection, submission and violence, which constitutes another particularly ambiguous form of trust based on personal relationship.

In Vale do Ribeira rural communities and in RAMA, self-production and family-level redistribution has largely ensured access to food in the context of social isolation and rising basic prices. This includes extended family, particularly in the case of the *quilombola* communities, which have also come together to respond to the public procurement of agricultural products (Food Acquisition Programme, PAA) launched by the federal government in its response to the threats to family farming and food security caused by the COVID-19. To these ends, these communities mobilized local organizations (*quilombola* associations), which is something that many rural districts could not do, in the absence of such a local political and trust basis. In some rural communities, emergencies also arose out of the suspension of access to public health services, when in March 2020 medical teams suddenly ceased their visits. Such issues were addressed either by having local elected representatives intervene, based on vertical, clientelist-type relations of protection, or by resorting to expensive private healthcare consultations (market-based). But often, these issues were not resolved at all. RAMA members shared a widespread feeling of powerlessness in relation to the pandemic, which pushed many of them to seek refuge in religious faith.

Overall, our observations suggest that, given the social marginality of the poor urban and rural communities in which AMESOL and RAMA members are embedded, increased protection needs arising from the COVID-19 pandemic have often been invisible or ignored by the state, reinforcing their position of subalternity. Local community responses have been mobilized in the face of this situation. These responses have been important, albeit sometimes insufficient or ambivalent, as to the type of protection they provide and the trust they are based upon. Vertical relationships of trust and protection, which build on and reinforce local hierarchies within local communities, are fundamentally different from the horizontal solidarity relations in AMESOL and RAMA. This difference explains the meaningfulness to the women of participating in these solidarity networks, where inequalities and discriminations are challenged. This difference also highlights the need for a careful analysis of the diversity of the types of trust based on personal relationships, especially in their degree of equality and their mutual interactions. Unequal relationships can be mutually reinforcing, just as egalitarian relationships can be. Egalitarian relationships can compensate for and sometimes transform unequal relationships, but they can also be excluded or distorted by them.

Right-based relations and the welfare system: trust and mistrust in governments

The position of subalternity of local communities in relation to the state and the limits of access to the welfare system needs to be understood in the context of trust and mistrust in institutions and the political class, which lies at the heart of the long ongoing political crisis in Brazil since 2013. The two terms of office of President Luís Inácio Lula da Silva (2003–2010) saw the introduction of a progressive political program, which benefited from a favorable international economic scenario and enabled improved social indicators and confidence in government. From 2013, the effects of the global financial crisis reached Brazil. The government of Dilma Rousseff (2011–2016) faced street protests against the high cost of living. These were led by right-wing movements calling for economic liberalism and accusing the president of corruption. Since 2014, political life has been punctuated by trials stemming from the gigantic police operation "Lava Jato". This involved the whole political class, pitting the judiciary against parliamentarians and the executive. Dilma Rousseff's impeachment and the 2016 parliamentary coup, followed by the conservative right-wing media campaign during Lula's 2018 trial, undermined Brazilian's trust in institutions and political parties, on both the left and the right. The ensuing polarization of Brazilian society explains the election of Jair Bolsonaro, whose authoritarian solution, based on the support of the armed forces and on presumed direct political action, bypassing the public institutions, was able to reassure part of the population, irrespective of social class (Feltran 2020).

The social protection system, with its links to the labor and financial (de)regulation model, has been at the heart of these disputes and their resultant crises of confidence in governments. President Lula's political path, "Lulism", took advantage of the favorable international climate, bringing together elements of neoliberal economic orthodoxy (inflation control, flexible exchange rates, primary budget surplus) with a left-wing agenda focused on reducing inequality (investing in social programs and infrastructure, making sustained minimum wage increases) (Singer 2009). These two combined antagonistic elements allowed him to reconcile class interests and to achieve a historic level of confidence of 81% of the population in 2010.[5]

In the context of democratization after the military dictatorship (1964–1985), the 1988 so-called "Citizens' Constitution" had established a public and universal health system (*Sistema Único de Saúde*, SUS). It was comprized of several levels of medical care and was funded by resources from the Union, the federated states and the municipalities. The socially minded action of Lula's government further stood out by bringing together several social programs into a large-scale conditional cash transfer program that gave priority to women, the *Bolsa Família*.[6] The management model for social programs during this period involved centralizing data on poor families into a single registry (*CadÚnico*) and decentralizing services at the municipal level, which could include the subcontracting of social organizations. The type of entry points for social policies across all the different territories has therefore varied greatly. On the one hand, this model was able to open spaces of facework commitment, for example through interdisciplinary medical teams, including community health agents. It could then create an embedded basis for trust relations and help extend the social protection system. On the other hand, this system may also have led to discretionary decisions by local agents, or even to the denial of access to care, such as reproductive health in units outsourced to certain religious institutions (Georges and Dos Santos 2016), resulting in exclusion and mistrust in social programs.

While these issues remained unresolved, the 2016 parliamentary coup suddenly shifted the debate to the deregulation of the labor market, and the drastic reduction of the budget for social policies. Michel Temer's government (2016–2018), in alliance with the conservative right, imposed an accelerated reform package including a freeze on social spending, an increase in the retirement age and labor market deregulation (Dari Krein, Gimenez and dos Santos 2018). These reforms were carried out in a climate of social tension between Michel Temer's unpopular government, which advocated for the measures in order to restore investor confidence and ensure economic recovery and social movements campaigning against the return of class politics and social exclusion. The arrival to power of Jair Bolsonaro shifted this debate to the field of authoritarian takeover, the role of the military and ultraliberal radicalization, including the privatization of education and health.

The Bolsonaro government's response to the COVID-19 pandemic falls under this ideological divergence and long-term power struggle. Equally, the government's position has rapidly evolved in recent months. At the pandemic's outset in March 2020, the president continued with arm wrestling other powers, calling for demonstrations for the closure of congress and the Federal Supreme Court, which had been investigating several charges against his sons and other close collaborators. He also claimed his priority was "the economy" and publicly criticized the social distancing measures taken by some state and municipal governors. A majority in congress disapproved of the president's position and endorsed a proposal for an emergency minimum income. This was supported by an extensive civil society network, denouncing the worsening of social and racial inequalities owing to the pandemic (Rede Brasileira de Renda Básica 2020). Bolsonaro finally passed the proposal, which entitled self-employed workers to R$600/month (around €100, doubled for single mothers who receive R$1,200/month), initially for a period of three months (April to June 2020), which was later extended until September, then December and then until 2021, covering an ever-smaller portion of the population with increasingly smaller amounts.

This aid has massively reduced the negative economic impact of the pandemic. In June 2020, the Brazilian Institute of Geography and Statistics estimated that 29.4 million households had had access to emergency aid, almost double the number of *Bolsa Família* beneficiaries (15 million registered in *CadÚnico*).[7] However, the Brazilian Basic Income Network drew attention to serious biases in its implementation 32.8 million were considered ineligible according to the government's data cross-checking methods. In a departure from previous governments' model of decentralized, *ad hoc* entry points to social aid in local territories, the aid was in fact implemented on the back of individualized computerized access, via an application requiring a smartphone or computer, internet access and an email account. The call center, which could have served as an alternative entry point, was overwhelmed and unreachable (Rede Brasileira de Renda Básica 2020).

Our interviews with RAMA and AMESOL women highlighted the difficulties people who were not already registered in *CadÚnico* have had in accessing the emergency aid. One young woman, a high school teacher living in a rural community where RAMA has a base, described the journeys she had to make to access the internet in this remote rural area, the incomprehensible errors sent back by the application when trying to register members of her community and her repeatedly unanswered phone calls to the call center. The women of AMESOL exchanged endless messages on their WhatsApp group in an attempt to work out what was true or false when it came to eligibility for aid, in the face of a profusion of fake news on social networks, fueled by vague government communication. RAMA members who finally received the bond waited in huge queues at the municipality's only point of withdrawal, which in several cases ended up with cash running out. Family, community and women's networks such as AMESOL and RAMA have tried to minimally re-embedded access to the scheme by exchanging information and advice, or even registering people onto the application. Inherent limitations to the scheme were an absence of intermediation owing to the individualized, computerized process, as well as uncertainty over eligibility, deadlines and cash withdrawal processes. In Giddens's terms, this is an excessively disembedded scheme, which has limited trust and the positive impact of the cash transfers. A key question is whether this disembeddedness of emergency aid is a dysfunction stemming from the urgency of its implementation, or if it represents a device to control the access of population to social assistance that sets up a new boundary to inclusion in social protection.

Other difficulties concerned access to the healthcare system in those rural RAMA communities where doctors' visits were abruptly interrupted in March 2020. On the outskirts of São Paulo, AMESOL women found themselves standing in front of health centers that were closed during their supposed opening hours, without information. These various difficulties had a common cause: a lack of established, functional spaces for intermediation. The consequence is a loss of confidence in institutions and governments.

An August 2020 opinion poll showed a roughly 5% rise in confidence in President Bolsonaro: 22% stated that they always trust him, 35% sometimes and 41% never (Datafolha 2020). The emergency aid program that the president had originally opposed, and which had enabled a temporary yet rapid fall in the poverty index,[8] certainly explains much of this renewed confidence. Ten days after the poll, the president stood up to the ultraliberal wing of his government and announced the replacement of the *Bolsa Família* and other social programs with a single, comprehensive program called *Renda Brasil* which, as of the end of 2021, still shows no indication of how it will be implemented. Whatever the outcome of the broader debate on a new design of social programs, it seems clear from the analysis of the president's discourse and action since the beginning of his term of office and of the pandemic, that his sudden position in favor of aid has been a case of political opportunism aimed to re-establish a basis of trust that is key to his own political survival, rather than a commitment to social inclusion.

Conclusion

Our analysis of trust, solidarity and protection sheds light on the social transformations brought about by the COVID-19 pandemic and the issues that are emerging for the period to come. The two subaltern women's networks analyzed here illustrate a singular type of trust based on feminist solidarity economy as a project for social transformation, and in its progressive implementation. Trust here is both political and pragmatic, and is based on personal relationships within each network, and with SOF staff and political allies in a network of social movements. This construction has proven resilient throughout the COVID-19 pandemic, thanks to the previously established trust and solidarity relationships and to wider use of virtual communication tools. This has enabled rapid responses, allowing for an adjustment of individual and collective economic activity and solidarity-based mutual aid actions. Virtual contacts have substituted face-to-face contacts in the context of social isolation, and allowed for solidarity relationships to be extended, to face the risks and handle the needs thrown up by the pandemic. In this sense, virtual contacts have played a key role renewing the pragmatic dimension of trust. However, the virtual elimination of face-to-face contact also weakened the personal basis and the political dimension of trust and is therefore not conceivable as sustainable over the long term.

Trust in solidarity networks is important from a theoretical and political viewpoint. It is as different from trust in abstract systems and in personal relations of friendships and sexual intimacy in "modern cultures" as it is from the "pre-modern" systems of trust based on kinship and community relations, as discussed by Anthony Giddens. As critical currents of feminism (Lugones 2007; Federic, 2012) and Modernity-Coloniality (Escobar 2003) have theorized, modernity implies the inclusion of certain social groups in world capitalism and its associated social systems, to the exclusion of others. For those outside this boundary, modernity means fragile or non-existent access to right-based welfare programs, and a need for relationships of trust and forms of protection complementary or alternative to state programs.

Our review of Brazil's political and social protection history, from Lula's government to Jair Bolsonaro's, in the context of a growing polarization of Brazilian society, illustrates the close links between level of trust in government, the welfare system and social inclusion. With the COVID-19 pandemic, Jair Bolsonaro's government experienced the renewal of the population's confidence due to its provision of emergency aid. However, it relied on a digital, dehumanized system of access to that aid which set up a series of barriers, clearly illustrating the limits to trust in an abstract protection system not embedded in social relations. Nor has this emergency aid changed the profoundly unequal structure of Brazilian society and the deficit of the state in poor territories.

In the otherwise highly diverse local communities where RAMA and AMESOL's women live, populations' vital needs are not being recognized by the state, reproducing a historical relationship of subalternity. Various forms of local protection based on personal relationships ranging from solidarity to the reproduction of social hierarchies or even submission to violence, offer responses to these vital needs. There is, as such, the need for careful analysis of these relationships, to recognize their importance while avoiding romanticizing them. It is to escape oppressive forms of local protection and to fill the void left by the state that the women of RAMA and AMESOL take part in solidarity networks that cultivate another, more egalitarian type of trust relationship.

Political and pragmatic trust in solidarity networks, trust in diverse personal relations in local communities and trust in the state-provided welfare systems are not mutually exclusive. They coexist in the lives and livelihood strategies of the people. In some cases, they are complementary, and in others they are contradictory toward one another. It would be a mistake to think that local and subaltern forms of trust are bound to disappear in global modernity. These forms constitute the ever-present reverse side of an unequal modernity. Given the crisis triggered in that modernity by the COVID-19 pandemic, they are playing an irreducible role in the resilience of excluded populations, and in the practice and imagination of other forms of trust, other economies and ways of life.

Notes

1 Isabelle Hillenkamp, corresponding author.
2 Available in French ("Les cultures des femmes. L'agroécologie face à la pandémie au Brésil" [Women's crops. Agroecology and the pandemic in Brazil], https://www.youtube.com/watch?v=Xhacr-xIrPc&t=3s) and in Portuguese ("As culturas das mulheres. Agroecologia face à pandemia no Brasil", https://www.youtube.com/watch?v=qGoOKNfe4MQ).
3 The names used are aliases.
4 See the investigative report in Portuguese "PCC, a irmandade dos crimonosos" (PCC [First Capital Commando], the brotherhood of criminals) by Naiara Galarraga Gortázar, Gil Alessi, published by *El Pais Brasil*, June 12, 2020, https://brasil.elpais.com/brasil/2020-06-12/pcc-a-irmandade-dos-criminosos.html (accessed on December 2, 2020).
5 According to a survey by the Brazilian Institute of Public Opinion and Statistics IBOPE in December 2010. Other surveys conducted during the same period reached similar results.
6 The programme's goal of covering 11 million households was achieved in 2006 (Pero 2012); 92% of the holders are women (2016 figures).
7 https ://agenciadenoticias.ibge.gov.br/agencia-noticias/2012-agencia-de-noticias/noticias/28354-distribuicao-de-auxilio-emergencial-alcanca-29-4-milhoes-de-domicilios-em-junho.
8 A study by the Brazilian Institute of Economy of the Fundation Getulio Vargas found that the extreme poverty index fell from 5% to 3.5% in May 2020, dropping to its lowest level in 40 years (https://blogdoibre.fgv.br/posts/auxilio-emergencial-faz-pobreza-cair-em-plena-pandemia).

References

Bernini, Carina Inserra. 2015. "*A Produção da 'Natureza Conservada' na Sociedade Moderna: Uma análise do Mosaico do Jacupiranga, Vale do Ribeira-SP*." PhD diss., University of São Paulo.

Butto Zarzar, Andrea Lorena. 2017. "*Movimentos sociais de mulheres rurais no Brasil: a construção do sujeito feminista*." PhD diss., Federal University of Pernambuco.

Caldeira, Teresa P. do Rio. 2000. *Cidade de Muros: Crime, Segregação e Cidadania em São Paulo*. São Paulo: Editora 34, Edusp.

Costa, Joana Simões, Ana Luiza Neves de Holanda Barbosa, and Marcos Hecksher. 2021. *Desigualdades No Mercado De Trabalho E Pandemia Da Covid-19*. Brasilia: Instituto e Pesquisa Econômica Aplicada (IPEA), Texto para Discussão No. 2684.

Dari Krein, José, Denis Maracci Gimenez, and Anselmo Luis dos Santos, eds. 2018. *Dimensões críticas da reforma trabalhista no Brasil*. Campinas: Curt Nimuendajú.

Datafolha Instituto dc pesquisa. 2020. *Avaliação do presidente Jair Bolsonaro. 11 e 12 de agosto 2020*. São Paulo: Folha de São Paulo, Datafolha.

Escobar, Arturo. 2003. "'Mundos y conocimientos de otro modo'. El programa de investigación de modernidad/colonialidad latinoamericano." *Tábula rasa* 1:51–86.

Fals Borda, Orlando. 1999. "Orígenes Universales y Retos Actuales de la IAP (Investigación Acción Participativa)." *Análisis político* 38: 73–89.

Federici, Silvia. 2012. *Revolution at point zero: Housework, reproduction, and feminist struggle*. Oakland, Brooklyn: PM Press, Common Notions.

Feltran, Gabriel de Santis. 2010. "Margens da política, fronteiras da violência: uma ação coletiva das periferias de São Paulo." *Lua Nova* 79:201–233.

Feltran, Gabriel de Santis. 2020. "'The revolution we are living.'" *HAU Journal of Ethnographic Theory* 10 (1). doi: 10.1086/708628.

Filho, França, Genauto Carvalho, Jean-Louis Laville, Magnen Jean-Philippe, and Alzira Medeiros. 2006. *Ação Pública E Economia Solidária – Uma Perspectiva Internacional*. Salvador, Porto Alegre: EDUFRGS/EDUFBA.

Fisher, Berenice, and Joan Tronto. 1990. "Toward a feminist theory of caring." In *Circles of Care: Work and Identity in Women's Lives*, edited by Emily Abel and Margaret Nelson, 35–62. Albany: Suny Press.

Franco, Maria Sylvia de Carvalho. 1997. *Homens livres na ordem escravocrata*. São Paulo: UNESP.

Fraser, Nancy. 1990. "Rethinking the public sphere: a contribution to the critique of actually existing democracy." *Social Text* (25/26):56–80.

Gênero e Número, and SOF. 2020. "Sem parar. O trabalho e a vida das mulheres na pandemia." mulheresnapandemia.sof.org.br.

Georges, Isabel, and Yumi Garcia Dos Santos. 2016. *As "novas" políticas sociais brasileiras na saúde e na assistência : produção local do serviço e relações de gênero*. Belo Horizonte: Fino Traço.

Giddens, Anthony. 1990. *The Consequences of Modernity*. Cambridge: Polity.

Hillenkamp, Isabelle, and Natália Lobo. 2019. Jeunes femmes de la campagne traçant leur chemin : apprentissages d'une recherche-action / Mulheres jovens do campo traçando caminhos: aprendizados de uma "pesquisação". In *Relatório de pesquisa*. Paris, São Paulo: Institut de recherche pour le développement, SOF.

Hillenkamp, Isabelle, and Miriam Nobre. 2021. "Agroecology and feminism in Vale do Ribeira (Brazil): Towards more sustainable forms of reproducing life." In *Social Reproduction, Solidarity Economy, Feminisms and Democracy*, 211–236. London, New York: Palgrave MacMillan.

Jalil, Laeticia. 2013. "*As Flores e os Frutos da luta: O significado da organização e da participação política para as Mulheres Trabalhadoras Rurais*". PhD diss., Federal Rural University of Rio de Janeiro.

Lucas dos Santos, Luciane. 2018. "When the domestic is also political: redistribution by women from the South. A feminist approach." In 3rd EMES-Polanyi Conference, Roskylde, Denmark: University of Roskylde, 16-17 April 2018.

Lugones, Maria. 2007. "Heterosexualism and the colonial/modern gender system." *Hypatia* 1 (22):186–219.

Masson, Dominique, and Janet Conway. 2017. "La Marche mondiale des femmes et la souveraineté alimentaire comme nouvel enjeu féministe." *Nouvelles Questions Féministes* 36 (1):32–47.

Mies, María. 1991. "Women's research or feminist research? (trad. esp. Investigación sobre las mujeres o investigación feminista? El debate en torno a la ciencia y la metodología feministas)." In *Beyond Methodology. Feminist Scholarship As Lived*

Research, edited by Mary Margaret Fonow and Judith A. Cook, 63–102. Bloomington: Indiana University Press.

de Oliveira, Dayse Maria da Silva Caciano, Douglas Ribeiro Barboza, and Paulo Roberto Raposo Alentejano. 2020. "Hegemonia do agronegócio e aceleração da contrarreforma agrária: as políticas do governo Bolsonaro para o campo." In *Políticas regressivas e ataques aos direitos sociais no Brasil: dilemas atuais em um país de capitalismo dependente*, edited by Larissa Dahmer Pereira and Douglas Ribeiro Barboza, 131–166. Uberlândia / Minas Gerais: Navegando Publicações.

Pero, Valéria. 2012. Bolsa Família : une nouvelle génération de programmes sociaux au Brésil. *CERISCOPE Pauvreté.* http://ceriscope.sciences-po.fr/pauvrete/content/part4/bolsa-familia-une-nouvelle-generation-de-programmes-sociaux-au-bresil?page=show.

Rede Brasileira de Renda Básica. 2020. "Problemas centrais na implementação do auxílio emergencial". In Texto para discussão 4–2020. www.rendabasica.com.br.

Saffioti, Heleieth. 2004. *Gênero, patriarcado, violência*. São Paulo: Editora Fundação Perseu Abramo.

Scherer-Warren, Ilse. 2008. "Redes de movimentos sociais na América latina - caminhos para uma política emancipatória?" *Caderno CRH, Salvador* 21 (54):505–517.

Schwenck, Beatriz. 2019. "Solidariedade e a vida das mulheres na Grande São Paulo: A experiência da Associação de Mulheres na Economia Solidária do estado de São Paulo, Brasil." *Otra Economía* 12 (22):120–132.

da Silva, Silvane Aparecida. 2019. "*O protagonismo das mulheres quilombolas na luta por direitos em comunidades do Estado de São Paulo (1988–2018)*". PhD diss., Pontifícia Universidade Católica de São Paulo.

Singer, André. 2009. "Raízes Sociais E Ideológicas Do Lulismo." *Novos estudos* 85: 83–102.

Spivak, Gayatri. 1988. "Can the subaltern speak?" In *Marxism and the Interpretation of Culture*, edited by Cary Nelson and Larry Grossberg, 271–313. Urbana, Chicago: University of Illinois Press.

Zaluar, Alba. 2004. *Integração perversa: pobreza e tráfico de drogas*. Rio de Janeiro: FGV Editora.

7 Trust in business in times of COVID-19

The case of the Aubervilliers garment wholesale market

Gilles Guiheux

> *The customer, if they know us, knows our qualities. They know the products. They trust us.*
>
> A wholesale dealer, October 2020

On January 23, 2020, owing to the rapid spreading of the COVID-19 virus, the city of Wuhan was put under quarantine by the Chinese central government. The following day, thousands of miles away, in Europe, France revealed its first three cases. These concerned a Frenchman of Chinese origin and two Chinese tourists who had stayed in the capital of the Hubei province where the pandemic started. By the end of the month, 100 people were infected with the virus in France. On March 11, the World Health Organization (WHO) declared the coronavirus epidemic a global pandemic. The following day, French President Emmanuel Macron spoke of "the most serious health crisis in a century" and decided to close nurseries, schools, colleges and universities. By March 15, the country had 5,423 confirmed cases, including 400 serious cases and 127 deaths. At noon on March 17, a general lockdown came into effect. All travel was to be reduced to the bare minimum; offices were closed, along with non-essential shops, and family and friends were prohibited from getting together until further notice. This initial lockdown would last 55 days, until May 11, and would be followed by two other milder ones in November 2020 and April 2021. During the pandemic, everyone became fearful of contact with objects and other people, including relatives, friends and colleagues. Citizens questioned public health policies and challenged political leaders and institutions. The event revealed, in a negative way, just how important a role trust plays, in normal times, in our relationship with the world.

Social sciences have paid increased attention to the issue of trust. George Simmel was one of the first to underline that trust is a major feature of modern societies. According to him,

> our modern life is based, to a much larger extent than is usually realised, upon our faith in the honesty of others (…) [We] base our gravest decisions on a complex system of conceptions, most of which presuppose the confidence that we will not be betrayed.
>
> (Simmel 1964, 313)

DOI: 10.4324/9781003291220-7

Simmel notably had in mind the need for confidence and trust when it came to carrying out business transactions. Since partners never know everything about their counterparts, there is always a certain degree of uncertainty that can only be overcome by trust. In traditional societies, both buyer and seller had personal knowledge of each other, as a result of which there was a certain sense of confidence. In modern societies, confidence is based on non-personal information and institutions, such as laws, contracts and other devices; confidence is "depersonalised" (Sellerberg 1982). As a result, when it comes to executing business transactions in developed industrial societies, reliance is based to a much lesser extent on personal trust and more on institutional conditions. The history of trust is a process of formalization, from trust limited to a community and individuals who know one another personally to trust among strangers based on regulations and rules or legally binding contracts.

Niklas Luhman has underlined how trust forms the basis of social order in a world that is getting increasingly complex; "without trust, one would not even be able to get out of bed in the morning" (Luhman 1968, 1). He sees trust as a mechanism for reducing the complexity required for the formation and stabilization of social order. Trust serves as an elementary mechanism for stabilizing expectations and thus as a condition of possibility for individual action. By reducing uncertainty and complexity, trust forms a routine background for everyday interaction that makes the social world predictable and reliable. Niklas Luhman extends Simmel's analyses with a systemic interpretation. Today's highly complex and differentiated society requires trust in systems such as money and power. According to him, it is the trust in systems that best manifests the contingency and the risk of modernity. In modern society, the spread of systemic trust does not make personal trust less important. Even the most bureaucratic organizations require trust in people.

When it comes to business, trust can be defined as "the information and reliability that enables two or more parties to coordinate, or to do business while having confidence in fair dealing" (Henderson and Churi 2019, 22). Trust, which facilitates exchanges, is at the same time an investment and a process. In a highly competitive market, social capital based on trust can be used to limit competition. It

> is like "ordinary" physical or financial capital in the sense that it requires investment, in the sense of sacrifice and effort, to build up, and when not maintained may deteriorate in time. Like physical capital, social capital is both the result of investment and a cause of economic performance.
>
> (Nooteboom 2007, 33)

Trust is also a process. Initially, when sellers and buyers have no knowledge of each other, their relationship is opportunistic, and risk has to be minimized by keeping orders small, then the business relationship gradually develops into a form of trust that allows for larger orders to be placed. As Nooteboom (2007, 43–44) puts it, the relationship starts "with minor transactions in which little trust is required because little risk is involved and in which partners can prove their trustworthincss, enabling them to expand their relationship and engage in more major transactions". Sellers need to put time and energy into earning their buyers' trust. Corporate brands, a topic extensively researched by the marketing literature, are one of the tools available to help develop trust between stakeholders.

Since the beginning of the 21st century, new technologies have led to the rapid digitization of economies. Exchanging goods and services via the Internet is based on *de facto* strangers interacting with each other. Nevertheless, in the online economy, just as in offline business settings, the presence of trust is a major precondition for successful transactions. This issue has been the subject of specific focus in management studies that have sought to assess how trust is being fostered in new and innovative ways (Henderson and Salen 2019). Looking specifically at the sharing economy, Mohlmann and Geissinger (2018) argue that, in peer-to-peer contexts, trust is built between strangers through the use of trust-enhancing digital cues. Confidence and trust in total strangers who have never met in real life is made possible by a trust-building process. Peer ratings, reviews, connections between peers' profiles with other social media networks, pieces of information such as name, age, particular skills, fields of expertise and general interests are among the cues that facilitate trustworthiness and trust between people without the mediation of institutional trust built either by governments or corporations (Mazzella et al. 2016). Does the digitization of economies mean that we are entering a new era of mutual trust? The rapid development of the sharing economy suggests the emergence of platform-mediated trust between peers (Sundararajan 2016).

This chapter aims at providing an answer to the question of trust in business and what it means in modern society. It is based on the empirical study of a wholesale market located in Paris (France). Interviews were carried out with four businessmen and four businesswomen involved in the garment sector and were focused on how respondents had adjusted their business practices due to COVID-19. The survey was carried out in October 2020, on the eve of the arrival of the second wave of the pandemic and before the implementation of the second lockdown. Six of the respondents in our sample were first-generation migrants in their 40s and 50s and two were second-generation, born and raised in Paris and having attended local business schools before inheriting their parents' garment businesses. Interviews lasted from half to over an hour. Contact was made by means of mutual acquaintances and notably through the leader of a federation of local Chinese associations.

The focus of the survey was on economic sociology. According to liberal economic theory, social actors participate in market exchange out of self-interest, and the coordination of economic activities through markets leads to an efficient allocation of economic resources. From a sociological perspective, individual actions must be understood within their social contexts. Embeddedness (Granovetter 1985) has become an established concept for describing the ordering processes that lead to a reduction of uncertainty and the social structuring of decisions in markets. Mark Granovetter (1985, 2005) notably points to the significance of network structures in the development of trust between market parties. As Jens Beckert puts it,

> a person who has already had positive experiences with an exchange partner in previous transactions or at least knows a trustworthy person who has had interactions with him or her is more likely to accept the contract risk than an

> individual for whom the exchange partner is a complete stranger. Networks through which information travels more easily are better equipped to induce cooperative behaviour because their structures facilitate the sanctioning of defectors.
>
> (Beckert 2009, 260)

Following this approach, we will pay attention to the different types of networks business dealers are embedded in, trying to assess how, at a time when social contact is reduced to a minimum, social and personal relationships still shape market transactions.

The chapter starts with an introduction to the wholesale market. The second part looks at how social relationships have been deeply affected by the pandemic. It ends with an analysis of the strategies developed by business dealers to circumvent the constraints of the lockdown and the role of digitization.

Aubervilliers: a Chinese wholesalers' district

History of the market

Aubervilliers is a city situated in the Parisian suburbs, at the junction of multiple transport routes. Bordered by several motorways, it is located between the *Périphérique* ring road that circles the French capital to the south, and the more recent A86 circular motorway slightly further away to the north. It is also east of the northbound highway leading to Charles de Gaulle (CDG) airport, less than half an hour's drive away is the north of France and beyond the Channel tunnel, Belgium and the Netherlands. Additionally, it is very well served by public transport, including two metro lines (7 and 12), two electric tramway lines and two regional express train lines (B and K).

As is the case in most northern Parisian suburbs, the economy was based mostly on industry, notably the chemical industry and warehouses, because the city is also crossed by the Saint-Denis canal (opened in 1821), on which goods could be transported to Paris's city center; the canal played a major role in the industrialization of Aubervilliers in the 19th century. In the 1960s, polluting industries moved out and the logistics sector needed more convenient facilities; as a result of which the whole Parisian region gradually shifted to the services sector. The city went through a period of economic decline, with many industrial buildings and plots of land lying empty. It is only during the last 20 years that the area has been developed into a network of wholesale markets, with Chinese traders selling mostly garment products but also shoes and small commodities.

The marketplace developed in three phases (Chuang 2018). Paris's garment district was originally located in the Sentier in the 2nd *arrondissement* and operated by businesspeople of Jewish origin, but the area gradually declined in the 1980s as rents increased and Chinese workers and bosses entered the sector. The garment district then moved to Paris's 11th *arrondissement*. In the late-1990s, owing to the continuous gentrification of the city center, a few individual business operators started to settle in Aubervilliers, attracted by the low cost of land and premises. In the mid-2000s, a few bold real-estate investors bought empty warehouses and converted them into collections of showrooms. Garment operators followed and rented these shops. The convenience of the new location compared to the congested streets of inner Paris contributed to the success of the project. Operating in Aubervilliers was much easier in a sector that constantly needed to load and unload goods arriving from suppliers and leaving for customers. There was also an obvious interest in concentrating all supply and demand in the same location to enhance competition and reduce the cost related to transport, packaging and handling. The third phase consisted of real-estate developers, including wealthy Chinese businessmen, deciding to develop brand new commercial centers dedicated to wholesale. In 2006, the CIFA Centre opened with 250 shops, while the Fashion Centre was inaugurated in 2015, boasting 310 shops on three levels and spanning a total of 55,000m,[2] promoting itself as Europe's largest commercial platform of imported products from China.

A former industrial city, Aubervilliers is now home to more than 1,000 wholesale dealers, most of them originating from the Wenzhou region of China's Zhejiang province. Investors and business operators were not the only players facilitating this transformation, as the city's local government decided to actively promote Aubervilliers as a Sino-French commercial platform, and more generally as a global city. The aim of the local government was to raise the international profile of the city, capitalizing on its history of immigration (Chuang and Trémon 2013, 190). According to Chuang Ya-han (2018), the development of wholesale activity gave rise to a growth alliance between the business operators, real-estate investors, developers and local government, all sharing a common interest in promoting urban renewal and the integration of Aubervilliers into the global economy.

A wide variety of market professionals

Today, as a global trade center, the city hosts all kinds of market professionals "whose task is to 'work on the market', i.e. construct it, move it, organise it, manage and control it, in short 'agencing' transactions" (Cochoy and Dubussion-Quellier 2013, 4). Besides shop operators, most of whom rent their premises, there are their employees, whether salespeole or manual workers loading and unloading goods. Most shops are actually operated by married couples. There are freight companies in charge of transporting the goods. There are insurance companies. There are banks and currency exchange businesses targeting foreign customers. There are packaging companies. There are design companies for those operators who would like to have their products designed in Paris while the goods are produced elsewhere. There are employment agencies. There are traders' associations. There are also hotels and restaurants serving the continuous flow of people visiting the markets.

There are different types of wholesale market. Some are housed in former industrial buildings and warehouses, while others, as mentioned, are located in brand new buildings built for this purpose. In the case of the latter, showrooms are arranged by product type, which makes it easier for customers to compare quality and prices. Since they are shaping economic exchanges, the markets can be considered as devices for constructing and organizing transactions.

The market professionals we interviewed are intermediaries between manufacturers and retailers. The manufacturers are, in most cases, based in Mainland China but also in the Prato region of Italy, where there is a cluster of textile Chinese factories, most business owners having come from Wenzhou and flocking to Prato in the mid-1990s to work in Italian-owned textile factories, where they quickly mastered the entire production chain. There are still a few businesses manufacturing in Paris but they are marginal. Wholesale traders travel to China twice to four times a year – once per season – to visit their suppliers for several weeks at a time. Those sourcing in Italy visit on a much more regular basis, sometimes as often as once a month on weekends, when the Aubervilliers shops are closed. Orders placed in China are much larger (thousands of pieces) than those placed in Italy (sometimes less than one hundred pieces); in the case of the former, goods take several weeks to arrive, whereas it takes only a few days from Prato. While Chinese products are cheaper, the risk is higher for the wholesaler, who has to place a large order before knowing if the products will meet the demand on the market. With Italy, products can be first tested on the market and if the product is successful, restocking takes only 24 to 48 hours, thus minimizing the risk through small orders and low stock levels (interviews).

Customers in Aubervilliers are French and European retailers coming from Belgium, the Netherlands, Germany, Poland, the United Kingdom, Spain and Portugal. They operate small stores competing with chain stores owned by international brands such as Zara and H&M, companies that source directly from producers in China and elsewhere. These retailers sell small quantities and don't have any knowledge of the production site. Some of these buyers in Aubervilliers are ethnic Chinese, in which case business transactions take place in Chinese. There are also African buyers for whom coming to the Paris wholesale markets is more convenient than traveling all the way to China.

Aubervilliers is a market where retailers source their products. It should be stressed that they buy from wholesalers in small quantities. They might order dozens or hundreds of the same item at a time, and if this item sells well, they will restock from the same wholesaler. In this economic system that includes producers, wholesalers and retailers, the economic risk is mostly taken by the wholesaler who buys the garments ahead of the season and runs the risk of not being able to sell his/her stock. A successful wholesaler is one who has a portfolio of regular clients whose needs he/she is familiar with; retailers have skills inherent in their human capital – the knowledge of their customers' requirements.

The need for trust and personal relationships

The Aubervilliers markets apparently make for the almost perfect scenario, since they encompass the three features of pure competition referred to in neo-classical economic theory. First, there is atomicity on both the supply and demand sides. The number of buyers and sellers is very large and none of the agents has sufficient weight to influence prices. For buyers, Aubervilliers makes it possible to consult a wide variety of product offerings in a very short space and time. There is also atomicity on the supply side, since a given wholesaler will specialize in one type of clothing – ladies'/men's/kids' wear, dresses, trousers or blouses, etc. – and will not be able to meet all of the needs of one particular customer. Secondly, products are largely homogenous. Garments sold on the market are very similar in quality and characteristics, and therefore almost interchangeable. These are cheap, low-end clothes that are often replaced because of fast-changing fashions. Aubervilliers is the home of cheap, fast fashion bought in small quantities. Finally, there is the fluidity, with free entry into and exit from the market. There are continuous incoming and outgoing traders. It is very easy to enter the market because of low barriers; a wholesaler just needs to rent premises and have a few contacts with garment manufacturers in China. And there are also many traders leaving the market at the same time because of the high level of competition.

In fact, the adjustment between supply and demand is not only undertaken through prices, but also through social relationships. Trust helps to reduce uncertainty, as highlighted by Simmel, who noted that it lies between complete knowledge and the absence of knowledge: "he who knows everything does not need to trust, he who knows nothing cannot reasonably trust" (Simmel 1999, 356).

In the wholesale market, information is asymmetrical and controlled by the seller. Garments are simple products and the possibilities for withholding information are limited as defects are visible, provided you can see and touch the product, which has not been possible during the pandemic. Still, the wholesaler can choose, in his or her own interest, not to reveal certain information regarding the production process in China or Italy to the potential buyer. For would-be buyers, the multitude of operators selling comparable products is also a puzzle. In such cases, to help deal with the opacity of the market, Lucien Karpick (1996) has shown that there are usually "arrangements for judgments". Trade names, product rankings and guides are all examples of impersonal arrangements. There are none in Aubervilliers. When it comes to labels, products carry the name of either the producer in China, the Aubervilliers wholesaler or the end retailer. Products change several times a year and are not ranked, and there are no published guides to the hundreds of operators, either. One way for retailers to reduce uncertainty is to rely on personal arrangements.

On the wholesaler side, the risk lies in the potentially opportunistic behavior of buyers who might place an order and never come back, and trust is "a type of expectation that alleviates the fear that one's exchange partner will act opportunistically" (Bradach and Eccles 1989, 104). The products are largely homogeneous and competition is therefore very tough, so the development of personalized social relations is a way of limiting competition.

There is evidence that these relationships of trust exist. Wholesalers have both old regular customers and new occasional ones, and because the long-term nature of the wholesaler-retailer contractual relationship creates a reassuring familiarity and predictable behavior among exchange partners, wholesalers aim at increasing regular customers (interviews). It should also be underlined that the wholesalers have a limited number of regular suppliers either in China or Italy for the same reasons. Besides maintaining a consistent level of product quality, the only way to develop a long-term relationship with clients is by using social skills. Customer loyalty, which requires special care to ensure that the bond of trust created is never damaged – for fear of the lasting negative impact this could have – is a strategy that can help stabilize the market.

The Aubervilliers wholesale market is both an economic and a social device. It is an economic device where the supply meets the demand for cheap garment products largely manufactured in China, meeting the needs of small retailers competing with large international chain stores and concerned with keeping up with fast-changing fashion. The market is also a social device of mutual trust which regulates exchange, a matter of knowing who to contact for a particular type of product. While it may appear to be a free, highly competitive and opportunistic market, players in the market actually aim at limiting the number of partners they trade with.

In a world of uncertainty and interdependence, trust enables actions and reactions to be anticipated and makes trade possible. Trust is one of the ingredients of successful coordination and one of the foundations of commercial activity. In the next section, we will look at how trust and social relations in the marketplace have been affected by the pandemic.

Garment wholesaling during the pandemic

During the 2020 spring lockdown, with offices and non-essential shops closed, the Aubervilliers wholesale markets were also completely closed. This forced closure did not have a major impact on the survival of the wholesalers' economic activity because the French government took various measures to address the negative consequences of the restrictions and to prevent companies from going out of business. Firstly, it guaranteed up to 90% of an eligible loan with respect to up to €300 billion of loans granted to registered companies. Secondly, all businesses, regardless of size, were allowed to defer social security contributions and tax payments (such as corporate income tax) due in March, April and May 2020. Thirdly, the French State contributed up to 70% of the gross salary of each employee within a limit of 4.5 times the hourly minimum wage in the case of full unemployment.[1] Private companies were then able to temporarily close their businesses without having to lay off permanent staff and go bankrupt.

By mid-May 2020, the Aubervilliers wholesale markets were able to reopen, but commercial transactions took a while to recover. Wholesalers as well as retailers were facing a hard time selling the garments already in stock and were reluctant to restock. The first customers to come back were French because regulations could make traveling to Paris impossible, depending on the country of origin. Besides, a lack of knowledge regarding the spreading of the virus and the frequent changes in French health policy resulted in a general fear of catching the virus. Visitors to the markets were fewer and orders were scarce and smaller. "A customer who used to order once a week now orders only once a month", says Respondent 8. Interviewing wholesalers, we tried to assess how, in these circumstances, they managed to keep their business going.

The old way of doing business

The main challenge wholesalers faced was to try and maintain commercial relationships while customers were unable to visit. This is how Respondent 1, a young man in his late twenties operating a showroom in Aubervilliers, described how his parents, who started the garment wholesale business, still managed their relationships with their customers:

> My parents are still doing business the old-fashioned way. Back in the 2000s, customers from all over France would come to buy garments in Paris, in the Sentier, the 11th arrondissement, and later in Aubervilliers. (…) *My mother waited at her store for the customer to come by, place their order, and leave with their merchandise* (…) My mother's *old customers* (…) We have their addresses. Sometimes their phone numbers. But we are not able to write them, to call them to tell them that we have something new. We do not know how to do this. *Customers are expected to physically come to the store*. My parents do not know how to maintain the commercial link. Except for the long-time customer. Calling to say hello, they don't know how to do it in French. They can do it in Chinese. This is one of the reasons we tell our parents to retire.
>
> (Respondent 1)

Respondent 1 is pressing his parents to retire and the pandemic has strengthened his opinion that the way they operate is no longer appropriate. He makes a clear distinction between the occasional opportunistic customers who pass by, look at the products, place an order and leave and the regular ones with whom his parents maintain long-standing relationships. He suggests that most of these are ethnic Chinese citizens who are easy to communicate with using Mandarin or Wenzhou dialect and that his parents cannot extend their network beyond this. The challenge brought about by the pandemic is that of being able to maintain long-term commercial relationships at a time when it is difficult, if not impossible, to meet in person.

For several years now, new technological devices have made it possible for customers to place their orders without physical meetings, all of them making use of various apps such as WeChat and WhatsApp, but as Respondent 3 makes very clear, that is not enough. Garments may be low-tech products, but buyers still need to touch them in order to make a judgment on their quality:

> Customers do not come to meet us; they come to see the products *(他来不是为了和我们见面，是要看到货物), to see the quality, to touch*

> *the fabric (摸到看一下).* After purchasing the product, if it sells well, then they will be able to place new orders by phone and WhatsApp. For me it's the same – when I started, I wanted to see the products, see if the fabric was suitable. For a customer you don't already know, sending a photo is not enough for a first transaction. *To check that the product is of a good quality, and that it will be comfortable to wear, you have to experience it for yourself* (货好不好，穿在人身上是不是舒服的，要试一试感觉一下). (Respondent 3)

Repeat orders can be placed remotely, but customers need first-hand experience of the product. This explains why retailers still visit wholesale markets.

Initial measures before the lockdown

At the beginning of 2020, most parts of French society remained largely indifferent to the health situation, but ethnic Chinese citizens were carefully monitoring the situation in Mainland China on a daily basis with great concern. Some of our respondents had traveled to their native country for Chinese New Year and shortened their stays. Fearing that his parents might catch the virus, Respondent 1 asked them to limit their commercial dealings to old and very familiar customers. At a time of fear, trust in business was limited to long-standing customers.

> By February, we were already worried. Then came the first cases in Italy. We [the two adult sons] told our parents they had to close the store. My mother had to make a trip to Prato to restock. We told her not to go. We were already worried for her. We told our parents, "you can open the metal shutter, but you keep the glass door closed. *Only when a customer you already know shows up, do you open up, let them in, and they must leave as quickly as possible, so no new customers. Only old customers could enter. But they shouldn't stay too long in the store*". That was just before the lockdown.
>
> (Respondent 1)

For the same reason, while the French government was still maintaining that wearing masks was unnecessary, Chinese wholesalers were already implementing preventive health measures that would later become mandatory:

> *We started wearing masks as early as February* [2020]. Because we were wearing masks at the time, customers found it odd and felt we were sick. At the time, French government policy maintained that only sick people need wear masks, but we were looking at what was going on in China at the time, and the Chinese government was saying that wearing masks could prevent the virus, so we were already wearing them.
>
> (Respondent 6)

In France, as was the case in many other countries, the pandemic led to an increase in anti-Chinese and anti-Asian behaviors. During the first week of the pandemic, individuals perceived to be "Chinese" or "Asian" were associated with the coronavirus and consequently suffered from discrimination, unfair treatment and, in some cases, physical attacks (Attané et al. 2021; Wang et al. 2021). Discrimination against Chinese people mainly occurred in public spaces such as on public transport. The media also played an important role in establishing prejudices, suggesting, for instance, that the Chinese were responsible for the pandemic because of their poor hygiene or their exotic culinary habits (Wang et al. 2021, 6). During the first weeks of the pandemic, relying on information received from China through relatives or friends, ethnic Chinese citizens would wear masks in public spaces, which provoked negative reactions. When masks became compulsory for everyone, this was no longer an issue.

After the lockdown and the reopening of the markets, business owners had to implement the same preventive measures that had become compulsory in shops all over the country, with customers and salespeople required to wear masks, hand sanitizer to be made available to visitors at the entrance and a plexiglass wall installed to protect the cashier.

The digitization of commercial relationships

Since visitors to the markets were scarce, wholesalers relied more than ever on digital tools to keep in touch with customers. What is striking in the following testimony is that digital tools were used not only to place orders but also to keep social relationships alive:

> *We have fewer customers coming to the showroom, but they are placing orders remotely instead. We send the photos and they order online, via WhatsApp. It is less costly for them. There are fewer risks involved. Orders are also smaller.* It's not a big deal as long as you maintain the social link.
>
> (Respondent 7)

Of course, this strategy of sending pictures of new products to generate orders can only be successful with customers who are already familiar with the seller. The same respondent clearly states that the pandemic has caused a shift in business practices:

> As soon as we have new products, we send photos of them to the customer. If the customer is interested, we send more photos. *We get in touch with them. They don't come to us any more so now we have to contact them. We didn't contact the customer before, we didn't have this reflex.*
>
> (Respondent 7)

In the days before the pandemic, all socialization would take place on site, but the pandemic has meant that it has now moved online. Respondent 2 is at the head of a much larger business than the others, so it is not only photographs that he sends to known customers, but also videos:

> [because of COVID], we can no longer welcome customers to our showroom. We can no longer visit them (…) Normally, when the client visits us, we hand them a paper book presenting the collection. (…) The paper book is no longer enough, so *we make 15-minute videos of our collections. We invite our buyers to watch these videos. We send these videos to our customers.* Beautiful models, lively music, and the product references appear in captions.
>
> (Respondent 2)

Digitization is, of course, not a new phenomenon; wholesalers were already using digital tools before the pandemic. Most of them have their own, albeit basic, website and there are three online marketplaces that have been developed over the last few years to enhance business. Toplook, Efashion and Parisfashion[2] are three websites set up by young second-generation Chinese entrepreneurs operating in different languages (French, English, Spanish, Italian and German). Wholesalers rent a page on the websites in order to advertise their products, and orders can be placed through the platforms for a fee. Up until 2020, however, only a very small share of the turnover was generated through the platforms or the websites; they were not a central component of the business. These websites are simple marketplaces where buyers can find information on the products such as size and color, but limited information on technical characteristics, none on stock levels and next to nothing on the sellers themselves.

Respondent 8 clearly explained how physical and online exchanges complement one another:

> *The store is where we meet new customers. The platform is also more for new customers.* If they then want to place bigger orders, they can come to the store. *The website is also made for old customers who already know us.* They go to our website to see new products if they can't come to the store.
>
> (Respondent 8)

Retailers have to already know the wholesalers to go to their personal website, so it is actually used by old customers, whereas platforms are used to attract new customers. Customers on a platform are the equivalent of the occasional customer passing through the shop and placing a trial small order. Respondent 2 is very confident that physical and online social exchanges will still coexist in the near future:

> There will be some adjustment and the two will coexist. We are not currently allowed to travel. Our customers cannot come to us and we cannot visit our customers, so we don't (…) What happens in a real meeting? *You can't lie when you meet for real. Face to face, you can't lie. I can't say the fit is good or the fabric is soft if it isn't. This is how we build a relationship, through the*

> *quality of our exchanges (…) We want to make the digital experience as pleasant as possible. The digital world cannot replace a real meeting. It can facilitate certain situations*. Physical meetings bring something else to the table. The first thing we do when meeting with a new customer is show them videos that are made to be sent to remote buyers – an example of the complementarity between tools for remote sales and those for face-to-face sales. These videos are so well made that we show them to buyers when they visit us. Then we move on to the next step: *we touch the products; we circulate the products.*
>
> (Respondent 2)

Through online exchanges, there is the risk that the wholesaler might behave in an opportunistic way and deceive the customer about the size or quality of the product, since the customer is unable to see and touch the product in person. This is what Respondent 7 had to say on the matter:

> Before [the pandemic], we were not used to ordering from pictures, through WhatsApp. They are starting to get used to ordering through WhatsApp from a photo. It is certain that in the future they will visit less. Of course, *they will always have to come to see the merchandise, to touch it, to stay in touch.*
>
> (Respondent 7)

Digital exchanges will become more widespread in the future but will not eliminate physical meetings altogether. Digital devices can be used to lure in new customers and to maintain social links with regular ones, but meeting physically and touching the goods will always play an important role.

Conclusion

The chapter has looked at how the COVID-19 pandemic has transformed business relations in the specific case of the Aubervilliers marketplace from a micro-sociological perspective. The main consequence of the pandemic is the impossibility for retailers to meet with wholesalers and see the products, while conducting business online. Social distancing made contactless transactions and interaction a necessity and accelerated the digitization of business relationships, a phenomenon that was already under way.

The shift from in-person encounters to online exchanges has increased the uncertainty surrounding products, which can no longer be touched, and reinforced the asymmetrical distribution of information in favor of wholesalers at the expense of retailers. Under normal circumstances, the customer can touch the product and easily identify any defects and qualities. When doing business online, however, retailers are at the mercy of the wholesaler and their claims, but since textile products are appraised in a sensory way by sight and touch, respondents argue that there will still be a need for a place and time where sellers and buyers can meet. There will be still a need for a physical marketplace. Commercial relationships will be based on both in-person encounters and virtual exchanges.

Digitization is a way to both initiate and maintain a social relationship between suppliers and customers. Mobile phone apps, videos, online streaming, online marketplaces and online shops are some of the devices that support business relationships, but the tools used by Aubervilliers wholesalers remain, for the time being, somewhat primitive and are far less complex than those that allow exchanges on the global platforms of the sharing economy. Trust is still mainly developed on the basis of in-person meetings between buyers and sellers. The digital tools used by our respondents provide a minimum of information on both products and wholesalers and do not help to develop a sense of trust between strangers in the way that platforms are already able to. Trust in the Aubervilliers ready-to-wear market is still mainly built on in-person exchanges, with the digital relationship merely supplementing this.

Two hypotheses can be formulated for the near future; either the wholesalers of Aubervilliers will make their online purchasing sites more complex and add the trust-enhancing cues characteristic of the platform economy, meaning that the bulk of their trading activity may one day take place online, or the digital activity will only ever continue to complement in-person relationships. The continuation of the survey will make it possible to identify which of these two scenarios is more likely.

Notes

1 See https://www.gouvernement.fr/plan-de-soutien-des-mesures-d-urgence-economique-durant-le-confinement

2 https://www.toplook.com; https://www.efashion-paris.com; https://parisfashionshops.com.

References

Attané, Isabelle, Ya-Han Chuang, Aurélie Santos, Su Wang. 2021. "Immigrés et descendants d'immigrés chinois face à l'épidémie de Covid-19 en France : des appartenances malmenées" [Immigrants and descendants of Chinese immigrants facing the Covid-19 epidemic in France: abused belongings]. *Critique internationale*. 91: 137–159. doi: 10.3917/crii.091.0140.

Beckert, Jens. 2009. "The social order of markets". *Theory and Society* 38: 803–840. doi: 10.1007/s11186-008-9082-0.

Bradach, Jeffery L. and Robert G. Eccles 1989. "Price, authority, and trust: From ideal types to plural forms". *Annual Review of Sociology* 15: 97–118. doi: 10.1146/annurev.so.15.080189.000525.

Chuang, Ya-han. 2018, "Aubervilliers sur Wenzhou, ou la transformation du Grand Paris par les entrepreneurs chinois" [Aubervilliers on Wenzhou, or the transformation of Greater Paris by Chinese entrepreneurs]. *Hommes et migrations* 1320: 51–58. doi: 10.4000/hommesmigrations.4050.

Chuang, Ya-han and Anne-Christine Trémon. 2013. "Conflicts and narratives surrounding Chinese quarters in and around Paris", in *Chinatowns around the World*, edited by Wong Bernard P. and Tan Chee-Beng, 187–214. Leiden: Brill.

Cochoy, Franck and Sophie Dubuisson-Quellier. 2013. "The sociology of market work", *Economic Sociology-European Electronic Newsletter. Max Planck Institute for the Study of Societies* 15(1): 4–11.
Granovetter, Mark. 1985. "Economic action and social structure: The problem of embeddedness". *American Journal of Sociology* 91: 481–510. https://www.jstor.org/stable/2780199.
Granovetter, Mark. 2005. "The impact of social structure on economic outcomes". *Journal of Economic Perspectives*. 19: 33–50. doi:10.1257/0895330053147958
Henderson, M. Todd and Salen Churi. 2019. *The Trust Revolution: How the Digitalization of Trust Will Revolutionize Business and Government*. New York: Cambridge University Press.
Karpik, Lucien. 1996, "Dispositifs de confiance et engagements crédibles" [Arrangements of trust and credible commitments]. *Sociologie du travail* 38(4): 527–550.
Luhman, Nicklas. 1968. *Vertrauen: Ein Mechanismus der Reduktion sozialer Komplexität.* Stuttgart: Lucius & Lucius Verlagsgesellschaft.
Mazzella, Frédéric, Arun Sundararajan, Verena Butt D'Espous, Mareike Möhlmann. 2016. "How digital trust powers the sharing economy". *IESE Insight Third Quarter* 30: 24–31. doi: 10.15581/002.ART-2887
Möhlmann, Mareike, and AndreGeissinger a. 2018. "Trust in the sharing economy: Platform-mediated peer trust", in *The Cambridge Handbook of the Law of the Sharing Economy*, edited by Nestor M. Davidson, Michèle Finck, John J. Infranca, 27–37. doi: 10.1017/9781108255882.003
Nooteboom, Bart. 2007. "Social capital, institutions and trust." *Review of Social Economy* 65 (1): 29–53. doi: https://doi.org/10.1080/00346760601132154
Sellerberg, Ann-Mari. 1982. "On modern confidence". *Acta Sociologica* 25 (1): 39–48. doi: 10.1177/000169938202500103.
Simmel, Georges. 1964. *The Sociology of Georges Simmel*. New York: The Free Press.
Simmel, Georges. 1999. *Sociologie [Sociology]*. Paris: Presses Universitaires de France.
Sundararajan, Arun. 2016. *The Sharing Economy: The End of Employment and the Rise of Crowd-Based Capitalism*, Cambridge, MA: MIT Press.
Wang, Simeng, Xiabing Chen, Yong Li, Chloé Luu, Ran Yan and Francesco Madrisotti. 2021. "'I'm more afraid of racism than of the virus!': Racism awareness and resistance among Chinese migrants and their descendants in France during the Covid-19 pandemic". *European Societies*, *European Societies* 23: S721–S742. doi: 10.1080/14616696.2020.1836384.

8 Trust beyond binary choices

Belgian Chinese immigrants' localization of a "Chinese bubble" in the "Belgian bubble" in the COVID-19 pandemic

Jingjing Li and Ching Lin Pang

Introduction

Trust is fundamental in the making of society (Durkheim 1984; Arrow 1972; Coleman 1988; Luhmann 1979; Paxton 2007; Simmel 2004). Trust is a social glue (Paxton 2007), a source of social order (Parsons, 1937/1968) and efficient transactions (Coleman 1988). The global health crisis of the COVID-19 pandemic has led to societal and economic turbulence across the globe, jeopardizing the lives and livelihoods of millions of people. It also presents an unprecedented challenge to the issue of trust and immigrant communities. Trust shapes and is shaped by various factors and their interactions including, but not limited to, policy responses, geopolitical relations, citizen's risk and threat perceptions, economic impact and personal experiences of COVID-19 in complex ways. Understanding the dynamics of trust in the context of migration and the current pandemic, is fundamental in both migration and trust research. In this chapter, we explore the possible relationship between Chinese immigrants in Belgium and their trust to both their home and host country. We ask whether mainland China's experiences and restrictive approaches toward the pandemic made Belgian Chinese immigrants more responsive to restrictive actions, such as the ones taken in China. To what extent has this influenced their trust in the host country? What are their strategies during the pandemic? Is it a binary choice of trust between the home country or the host country?

Firstly, we present a literature review on trust research in the context of migration and the current COVID-19 pandemic. Secondly, we explain our research methodologies in studying trust and immigrant community before presenting our case study of a Chinese heritage school and its ten voluntary teachers, their perceptions of the "Belgian bubble" and the "Chinese bubble" in the third part. Fourthly, the Chinese heritage school is presented as a site where the localization of Chinese approaches in the Western context emerges. By examining the trust-dilemma and trust enactment of Chinese immigrants in Belgium encounter in the context of COVID-19 pandemic, this chapter answers the call to epistemological pluralism in understanding trust (Isaeva et al. 2015).

DOI: 10.4324/9781003291220-8

Trust research in the context of migration and the COVID-19 pandemic

International migration and trust have been debated by scholars to verify the origin of trust, in two main competing perspectives, the cultural versus the experiential dimension (Dinesen 2013; Dinesen and Hooghe 2010; Ljunge 2014; Dinesen and Sønderskov 2018; Moschion and Tabasso 2014; Nannestad et al. 2014; E. M. Uslaner 2008; Helliwell, Wang and Xu 2016; Wu 2020). The cultural theory of trust believes that trust is learned and imprinted in early life socialization and immersion in cultural and heritage context. Thus, it tends to remain rather stable over time with limited impact from changing environments (Wu 2020). Similarly, in international migration research, some scholars argue that immigrants, including recent immigrants and immigrant descendants from various ethnic backgrounds and geographical origins, tend to trust their country of origin or at least the country of origin plays a positive impact on their levels of trust, and that their trust does not adapt to the new environment and experiences (Ljunge 2014; Moschion and Tabasso 2014; E. M. Uslaner 2008; Bilodeau and White 2016; Rice and Feldman 1997; Soroka, Johnston and Banting 2007). The overall conclusion is that trust is cultural (Wu 2020). Alternatively, scholars from the experiential theory of trust associate trust with changing life experiences and circumstances within specific contexts. It is situated at different levels and subject to change (Glanville J.L. 2007; Hardin 2002; Rothstein and Uslaner 2005; Paxton and Glanville 2015; Dinesen and Hooghe 2010). In international migration, some scholars discovered migrants' trust has adapted to the trust level of the hosting country, including immigrants and emigrants (Abascal and Baldassarri 2015; Bauer 2015; Dinesen 2012a, 2012b; Dinesen and Hooghe 2010; Dinesen and Sønderskov 2018, 2015; Nannestad et al. 2014; Paxton 2007). Admittedly, these two perspectives of examining trust within the migration context have provided primary theoretical frameworks to explore the relationship between migration and trust. However, they are subject to changing and selecting immigrant policies of hosting countries (Wu 2020; Bilodeau and White 2016) and changing conditions of trust over time in countries of origin (Dinesen and Sønderskov 2018). Moreover variations in understandings and measurements of trust vary across cultures and societies are overlooked (Delhey, Newton and Welzel 2011; Fukuyama 1995; Simpson, McGrimmon and Irwin 2007), while hardly acknowledging impact from discriminatory experiences of the immigrants (Wu and Wilkes 2016). Therefore, comparing levels of immigrants' trust between their country of origin and their host country may be problematic, all the more as it implies a binary choice between trust toward either the host or the home country. Such a dichotomy fails to include the evolving relations of immigrants with host and home country, who may adopt a "both-ness" perspective. In so doing it overlooks immigrants' agencies and constructive capabilities to combine the best of "both worlds", especially in times of an unprecedented global health crisis.

Since the onset of the coronavirus pandemic studies on the influence of pandemic on trust have proliferated. Following abundant epidemiological, medical and virological studies, the primary research focus has been placed on the dynamic between trust and institutions, including but not limited to topics such as (positive and negative) correlation between social trust, risk management and institutional performance (Kye and Hwang 2020), relationship between (presence or absence of) trust and governmental policy responses (Devine et al. 2020), the interaction between public trust in government, risk management and risk communication (Wong and Jensen 2020; Balog-Way and McComas 2020; Longstaff and Yang 2008; van Dijck and Alinead 2020; Lovari 2020), impact of political standpoint, racial background, religious beliefs, social class and residential location on trust toward scientists (Evans and Hargittai 2020). Most, if not all, of this trust research relies mainly on surveys conducted with the national context. However, other relevant and equally critical research topics for public health such as the role and/or experiences of various types and groups of immigrants (Guadago 2020), who are disproportionately affected and possibly stigmatized and marginalized (Yoon, Feyissa and Suk 2021; Guadago 2020), have not yet fully researched. In this chapter, we bring the emergent discussions of migration and trust into conversation with the emerging body of literature on trust research in times of the COVID-19 pandemic. It is within this grand and critical context that we adopt an interpretivist, context-sensitive research perspective on trust (Isaeva et al. 2015) aiming to explore the messy "life-worlds" (Habermas and Stark 1988) of migrants' experiences during the pandemic. We bring the experience of Chinese immigrants in Belgium to the fore as an important stakeholder group in the COVID-19 crisis living in two worlds, while being confronted as "categorically untrustworthy" (Isaeva et al. 2015, 13) due to their ethnic background, especially in the early stage of the outbreak. We rely on an emic approach in examining their experiences based on the analytical concept of trust within a pandemic context. In this sense, trust is not universal and definitive (Bachmann 2011; Dietz 2011) nor is it a choice between home or host country but rather context-based and encompassing evolving practices and processes.

Research methods

How to measure trust has been a key topic of discussion in trust research (Tillmar 2012). The existing literature on measuring trust is largely based on standard survey, which might decrease the validity of the results (Devine et al. 2020). In fact, the multidimensional nature of trust requires methodological diversity (Isaeva et al. 2015) and plural measurement of trust beyond "binary choices" (Devine et al. 2020).

Tillmar (2012) proposed a combination of semi-structured interviews and ethnographic methods in her cross-cultural comparative research of trust. Inspired by this approach in conjunction with our longitudinal involvement and deep connections with the study site,[1] we combined onsite and online ethnographic fieldwork and in-depth interviews. The onsite fieldwork is conducted in a Chinese heritage school (hereafter referred to as CHS). Ten voluntary teachers participated in the research over a period from the start of the pandemic in January 2020 to early

November 2020 when Belgium implemented its second national lockdown, and later extended to the summer of 2021 when containment measures were loosened in Belgium. The term heritage school refers to immigrant heritage language school outside of the formal education system of the host society as a site of teaching immigrant languages and cultures, providing a social and emotional support system (Kim 2011), a crossroads of cultures, space for identity formation (Hsu, Pang and Haagdorens 2012) and diasporic subjectivity contestation (Doerr and Lee 2009). The onsite fieldwork allowed us to observe Chinese immigrants' responses to the pandemic and strategies when living in – and with – two worlds at the levels of the Chinese community and individuals. However, with the development of fieldwork as well as global spread and rapid evolving of COVID-19, our original intention was changed. we realized there seems to be a gap between the "European reality" (Kinnvall 2016) and the "Chinese reality" in responding to the pandemic. The balancing act between the two realms namely "the European/Belgium bubble" and the "Chinese bubble" takes place and gain prominence at the CHS where we observed a practice of localizing "Chinese bubble" in the context of the "Belgian bubble".

We also conducted ten in-depth semi-structured interviews with ten key interviewees working as voluntary Chinese teachers at the CHS in late October to early November 2020, using digital technologies particularly WeChat, a popular social media platform among Chinese, given the constraints presented by lockdown and other preventive measures. To respect the will and to protect the anonymity of the interviewees, we use numbers to refer to them. In total, we interviewed ten women who work as voluntary teachers at this CHS. We interviewed them based on their long-time (at least two years) involvement with the CHS, knowing they would have good knowledge and a long-term relationship with the CHS. The ten interviewees are all female because the schoolteachers are all female.[2] They are between 37 and 60 years of age. Nine come from Mainland China and one from Hong Kong. Their levels of education range from high school to bachelor's degree. Their professional occupations vary, including housewife (former bank clerk, tour guide), freelance interpreter, freelance architect, Chinese restaurant owner and employee in Belgian company. They are all first-generation immigrants settled in northern Belgium. Half of them are (or was) married to a non-Chinese spouse. Their main network varies. Some mainly interact with the local Chinese community, while others have interactions beyond the Chinese community. The interviews aimed at gauging their perceptions of home and host society during the global health crisis and their corresponding coping strategies. The semi-structured interviews revolved around four questions concering their perspectives and comments on government and public's responses to the pandemic in both host country and country of origin, namely Belgium and Mainland China, as well as their comments on the CHS's responses to the pandemic. Lastly, interviewees were invited to share personal emotions and feelings since the beginning of the pandemic in China until the time when the interviews took place. We implemented a narrative approach in these interviews because it allows the interviewees to freely share their ideas, both positive and negative, their personal stories and experiences, encouraging them to express emotions. In so doing, the interviewees can emphasize what they deem most important or hard to understand when facing the coronavirus pandemic, uninterrupted by external question. The interviews were taken at a convenient time for the participants. Each lasted from 30 minutes to 2 hours, varying in length because of the narrative nature of the approach. In a few cases, the participants added more information through voice messages after the interview. The interviews were taken in Chinese and were translated and analyzed by the authors. We acknowledge the formal and diplomatic style of speaking in the interviewees' responses during the interview. This could be led by two interlinked reasons. Firstly, the interviewees' role as (voluntary) Chinese teachers at CHS made them familiar with using formal and diplomatic language. Secondly, being interviewed in Chinese, their native language, facilitated the interviewees' use of classical and formal expressions. To deepen our understanding of trust with the interviewees in a natural setting, we contacted them in May and June 2021. These visits included participating two CHS online meetings and one onsite gathering in the CHS. On these occasions, casual talks were initiated with interviewees about their current attitudes and concerns about the containment measures and the ongoing vaccination program in Belgium. Fieldnotes were taken in these follow-up visits and analyzed.

In addition to the ethnographic method, we also conducted a critical reading of news reports on how the Belgian media report on China during the pandemic. We chose to analyze all articles of the daily newspaper *De Standaard*, considered as a reliable and informed news outlet between the period of January 1, 2020 and December 31, 2021. We used two search terms: "Corona and China" and "Corona and the Chinese" (www.standaard.be).

In what follows, we present the evolving social process of trust through the case study of Belgian Chinese immigrants' localizing a "Chinese bubble" in the context of the "Belgian bubble". The term "bubble" was inspired by the Dutch buzzword "knuffelcontact" (cuddle contact) with whom social distancing could be ignored during the pandemic. Belgium's National Security Council used "knuffelcontact" to indicate the number of people an individual or a household that are allowed to meet in specific situations to limit social contacts during the COVID-19 pandemic at different stages. The term "bubble" thus indicated a non-voluntary choice of – among our most intimate social relations – who can be trusted or distrusted, to maintain physical and intimate contact in times of uncertainty and ambiguity. Overtime we realized a seemingly gap between the "European reality" (Kinnvall 2016) and the "Chinese reality" in responding to the pandemic. At the same time, we observed how balancing acts between the two realms have taken place and gained prominence at the CHS in Belgium where Belgian Chinese immigrants have been localizing a "Chinese bubble" in the context of the "Belgium bubble". Within this context we extend the term "bubble" from its original use. The term "bubble" is not a process of "othering". Instead, it is a process where Belgian Chinese immigrants' trust, including trust in government and medical professionals, trust in institutions and social trust toward both China and Belgium evolve over time during the pandemic.

The "Belgian bubble"

The term "Belgian bubble" is used to represent the mutual gaze between societal groups within one country and between countries.

On the one hand, it refers to the Belgian public opinion toward Mainland China's early and subsequent reactions and containment policies to the COVID-19 pandemic as well as toward Chinese immigrant communities in Belgium. As for the Belgian gaze toward China and the Chinese community, there is a scarcity of academic data and reports. In the 2020 Annual Report Vulnerable Human Rights in Times of Crisis (2021) of UNIA, the interfederal institution promoting equal opportunities and fighting racism, there is no explicit mentioning of hate speech or other racist acts against the Chinese. In the media, however, there are several news items highlighting the rise of discrimination and racism toward Chinese and Asians. As for the general perception and representation of the pandemic in China the search term "Corona and China" for the period between 2020 and 2021 and in all categories of the newspaper *De Standaard* 812 results were yielded, of which only 70 articles discussed China and the pandemic. It should not come as a surprise that only 13 articles presented a positive view, whereas most of the articles were highly critical revolving about the origin of the virus, censorship toward critical journalists, Ai Weiwei's documentary on the pandemic, Taiwan's effective and transparent method, public shaming. As for the 13 positive articles, the content lauded the efficiency of the Chinese method, the rapid economic recovery, the discipline of the Chinese people. Even when China is presented in a positive way it usually comes with a warning. The heading "the best but also the worse comes from China" is one of these positive articles captures the ambiguity of the public opinion. It is also worth mentioning that two articles in mid-March 2020 when the country went into a comprehensive lockdown underlined the importance of the Belgian government support to local businesses and working population. The headings read as follows: "The economic support can never be too excessive" and "The day that the (government) budget becomes (for a little while) a side issue". For the search term "Corona and the Chinese", among the 141 results only 4 articles dealt with the eruption of discrimination and hostility toward the Chinese. Moreover it is important to note that the term Asian is more used than Chinese. The coverage of anti-Chinese sentiments is clearly less abundant than in other countries. There is no available data to confirm the hypotheses whether this was due to lesser discrimination or underreporting. However, the seemingly emergence of discrimination has triggered NGOs and Chinese individuals to launch campaigns and initiatives to render the anti-Chinese/Asian sentiments more visible. The main purpose is to debunk the notion of the Chinese/Asian as the model migrant by sharing migration and discrimination stories across generations and beyond the current COVID-19 period.

On the other hand, the "Belgian bubble" also refers to Belgian Chinese immigrants' perceptions of the "Belgian reality" during the COVID-19 pandemic, particularly from the Chinese immigrant females working as voluntary teachers in the CHS in relation to their perceptions of Belgian society's responses to the COVID-19 pandemic, including that of the government, the public and local schools during the entire period of the pandemic. Living in Belgium provided the Chinese female immigrants the chance to observe, compare, reflect and react on the responses and measures to contain the pandemic. Through their explanations and perspectives, they showed how they have engaged and disengaged with the local community during the pandemic at different stages. It is through their perceptions that we could grasp the evolving and changing process of trust and distrust afforded by the pandemic and their relation with the host society. In general they display mixed institutional trust toward Belgian authorities' responses to COVID-19 pandemic. On the one hand, as long-time residents in Belgium they understand the complexity and specificity of the Belgian political system and society. As a result, some are highly aware that a China-style lockdown policy was not possible to implement and showed pragmatic trust toward the host society's social assistance and labor system. Their trust is based on the governance and information capacity of the system and/or political leaders to make the best decision for the country. Interviewee 1 is a housewife and her family relies on social allowances due to work injuries of her husband. The system has been assisting the family for more than a decade. Based on the delivery of welfare services, she trusts the political authorities and system for practical reasons. She has defended Belgian authorities' implementation of a "soft lockdown":

> They (those who support fuller and stricter lockdown) don't care about the national economy. Those who make national decisions are evaluating the situation from the national perspective. For the sake of economy, they would not implement full lockdown. For people like my family, we rely on the (welfare) system therefore we hope the best for the system.
>
> (Interviewee 1)

For small-business owners such as Chinese restaurateurs, their institutional trust toward host country increases after receiving business support from different institutions during the pandemic. One interviewee shared her appreciations of the government's subsidies that helped her restaurant to survive the lockdown period:

> Before the pandemic, we were only busy with our own restaurant, never paid attention to policies. The pandemic brought catastrophic impact to my restaurant business. I am so grateful we received financial assistance from the government. It's very helpful for me. At least we could buy food to survive. It's been 8 months already. If the government didn't give us subsidies, we couldn't hold it together anymore. At least they give us a chance to breath. Besides the subsidies, they also contacted me and suggested me to attend training classes at VDAB (Flemish employment department). You know, to prepare for other employment chances in the future in case we need it. I am very happy about their suggestions. At least it means they care about us small-business owners.
>
> (Interviewee 8)

Trust here is a sense of confidence in the reliability of the system and the people operating this system based on their professional knowledge and governance capability, the full range of information being collected to enable decision making at a macro level for the long-term benefit of society. Some interviewees, espousing institutional trust choose to interpret the government' decisions regarding the pandemic from the macro level, or in their words "bigger picture". Conversely, others indicated a lack of "pragmatical trust" as the result of the institutional fragmentation of Belgium federal system where each level of government has its own respective competences which impedes a coordinated and rapid response.

> It's not easy, the Belgium case. There are federal, provincial and city government. It is already difficult to form a coalition government.[3] Let alone taking care of the COVID. We have 9 health ministers in Belgium! Too many voices.
>
> (Interviewee 4)

Interviewee 4 is a retired former Chinese restaurant owner who has lived in Belgium for more than five decades. In contrast, other interviewees displayed decreased levels of trust as a result of local authorities' slow responses, underestimation of the pandemic as "just like a flu" and downplayed the importance of wearing face masks, misleading information to the public, lack of supervision system on requested self-quarantine at home, and dereliction of duty from certain public figures.[4] Moreover, most of the interviewees criticized Belgium's general distrust toward China (geopolitical mistrust/distrust that are constantly presented in local media narrative) thus "was too arrogant to learn from China".

As for using face mask at the beginning of the outbreak, most interviewees revealed conflicting views. On the one hand, as Chinese migrants they learned from the Chinese experience the great significance of wearing face mask as a positive protective measure. On the other hand, Belgian health authorities were skeptical about the use of face masks at public spaces, which was stereotyped as a sign of sickness, thus causing social stigma and prejudice. The Belgian authorities prioritized other measures such as social distancing and hand hygiene. Globally, such underestimation of using face mask in the early stages of the pandemic has led to friction and discrimination toward Chinese and/or Asian migrants' everyday life (Ma and Zhan 2020). As a result, some interviewees felt fearful and had to device tactics to render the wearing of face mask less visible in daily outgoing:

> When I went to Lidl (supermarket), I put on scarf to cover the mask on my face. The government said it is not necessary. They created such an environment discouraging wearing a mask. For us (Chinese), it took a lot of courage to wear a mask (afraid of being publicly ostracized) in the public space.
>
> (Interviewee 5)

Furthermore, most interviewees deplored the impact of the Belgian media's general negative reports on China. Some condemned Belgium's refusal to acknowledge and learn from the effective measures taken in China in handling the pandemic, such as raising public awareness to use face mask in public spaces and informing the public about the seriousness of the coronavirus. Western media's general critical coverage of China led to an underestimation and slow response to the pandemic in the West, which could bring negative impact on mental health to immigrant individuals (Gao 2021). The following interview reflects this view:

> They (the Belgium authorities) are quite arrogant. Overall they distrust China. There is always negative information about China. In the Netherlands it is more open. They reported on Chinese tourists' domestic traveling during the National Holiday week (indicating positive image of China having taken the coronavirus condition under control). Here (in Belgium) they would never cover such positive news about China. Even if China has an effective vaccine, they (Belgium authorities) would not trust China. It's just a fact.
>
> (Interviewee 7)

Generally our interviewees have mixed perceptions toward the response to the COVID-19 pandemic of the Belgian authorities, including both positive trust attitudes as well as criticism and distrust. However, they all demonstrated certain degrees of understanding toward the complexity of the Belgian political system and the geographical specificity of Belgium as a transit country in the center of Europe which makes the Chinese model of strict lockdown and border control near impossible.

Mixed social trust

The host country's higher trust to its citizens for self-regulation – such as unsupervised self-quarantine and non-mandatory wearing of face mask in the early stage – was not shared by Chinese migrants. Instead they see a lack of self-regulation along the locals, especially youngsters, who responded to the pandemic in a careless, indifferent, irresponsible and self-centered way.

> I live in an apartment building. My neighbors are mostly elderly. They didn't wear a mask when going outside. I was so worried about them. My husband's colleagues were also very careless. They didn't follow the measures of home quarantine after traveling back from an Orange zone. They even visited their families and friends and did grocery shopping in supermarkets. I am speechless and furious about such people. I don't understand why the public is so at ease even when the daily infected cases reached more than 10,000. They lack the spirit of cooperation.
>
> (Interviewee 2)

While denouncing the individualistic behaviors of the locals, they nonetheless made efforts to make sense of their behaviors. Perhaps they were misled by the government, local media and even schools that downplayed the severity of the pandemic.

Another bone of contention, especially among Chinese immigrant parents was the unpreparedness and difficult transitioning to online education during the first lockdown. Notwithstanding the anxiety for infection and sickness, interviewees generally support the government policy to send school-age children back to school after the lockdown to avoid jeopardizing their education.

> Online teaching does not exist in elementary school. My son's school only sent out emails telling him to do the assignments. He had to rely purely on self-study. When he didn't understand something there was no instance he could turn to.. I wouldn't send my son to school during the pandemic, but I understand the policy (that pupils must attend school). I wouldn't risk my son's life to go to school but there is no other way! There is just no qualified online education!
>
> (Interviewee 10)

Against this context of mixed trust toward local institutions and society the Chinese immigrants developed their Chinese approach to the local environment, which can be framed as the "Chinese bubble".

The Chinese bubble

The "Chinese bubble" refers to Belgian Chinese immigrants' perceived "Chinese reality", reflecting their mixed approach toward the pandemic and their changing trust toward China's approach. Their perceptions of China's approaches to the pandemic has been subject to waves of trust and distrust. First the distrust and critique on the Chinese government in early 2020 has evolved into trust in China's restrictive measures since February 2020 and this trust has increased in March 2020 when Belgium became the epicenter of the pandemic. However this trust has lost its strength since June 2021 when they started to question China's zero tolerance policy.

In January 2020, our interviewees discussed their concerns based on the information they received from friends and families on WeChat about an unknown but highly infectious disease in Wuhan. During this conversation nine interviewees showed disappointment and criticism toward the Chinese government's non-reaction. They also showed deep concerns about a possible cover up of the problem, along with a relief that no families from their fellow colleagues were in Wuhan at the time, alongside empathy to the sufferings of people who were in Wuhan. This concern, if not yet distrust, intensified after attending the Chinese Spring Festival Parade in the Eastern Belgian city of Liège on January 18, 2020, where a group of dancers from Wuhan were invited to perform at the parade. In the subsequent days the proliferation and deepening of the anxiety and distress among the Belgian Chinese community prompted the Chinese Embassy in Belgium to respond. On Febraury 1, 2020 the Embassy provided the number of Wuhan visiting performers, their arrival and departure dates in Belgium and a statement on their health conditions. "All 21 visitors have safely passed the observation period. No one has showed flu or pneumonia-like symptoms including headache, fever, and coughing".[5] This did not fully stem the distress among our interviewees, especially after the death of doctor Li Wenliang in February 2020.

Over time, their trust toward the Chinese government has evolved positively with the implementation of strict nationwide containment measures (Liu, Yue and Tchounwou 2020). This may also be related to China's experiences in controlling the SARS virus in 2003 as interviewee six referred to. It also indicates the social trust toward Chinese citizens' collective efforts and compliance with the government's measures. At the time of our interviews in September and October 2020, all ten interviewees endorsed China's strict and preventive approaches, including that of governments and Chinese citizens. They spoke highly of China's responsive measures in controlling the pandemic. As this interviewee noted:

> China has taken it very seriously from the beginning. From the start, the government told the public to wear masks and keep social distancing. Chinese people are more conscious about the pandemic than people here (Belgium). We experienced SARS (in 2003), (therefore) we know how serious this can be. When the (Chinese) government warned (that) this time it could be worse than SARS, I know it's something very fearful coming.
>
> (interviewee 6)

Others praised Chinese citizens' compliance with Chinese government's prevention measures. Such collaboration was described by interviewee 10 as a "difference between collectivism and individualism", or as the following interviewee referred to as a "Chinese mindset":

> I have a mindset of China. I think it is important to cooperate with the government in the pandemic. China has taken the COVID-19 pandemic very seriously. Chinese have learned to take into consideration of others, not to bring trouble to others. I'd feel so guilty if I gave the virus to other people. It's a different mindset than here.
>
> (Interviewee 2)

Admittedly, the global reach of the pandemic has created some sort of competition among governments and their respective response to the pandemic. For Chinese migrants in Belgium, as in many other countries, they constantly observe and compare measures taken in China and their efficacy with those in Belgium. Needless to state that this comparison exerts a significant impact on their trust to both worlds. However, contrary to existing literature that presents a dualistic perspective on trust to either the home country or the host country, the Belgian Chinese community has attempted to adapt the Chinese approach to local Belgian context.

Despite the mixed approach of the Belgian Chinese community, they share commonalities with other Chinese communities in other countries. Unlike in many reported cases where immigrants' communities had higher risk of exposure and transmission due to their lack of awareness of local risk prevention measures, linguistic barriers and adherence to specific cultural customs and practices, barriers to access health care and crowded living conditions (Arfaat 2020; Greenaway et al. 2020), Chinese diaspora communities across the globe have taken early preventive actions including keeping physical distancing, mask wearing as well as stricter hand hygiene measures due to their familiar, cultural, social and economic ties with mainland China, Hong Kong and/or Taiwan (Roberts 2020; Krause and Bressan 2020). Some Chinese diaspora communities even made efforts to assist host society with preventive actions, and thus to some degree curbing the spreading of coronavirus in local host community, while influencing local political responses to the pandemic (Krause and Bressan 2020). In the Belgian context, all interviewees describe the local Chinese community's response to the pandemic as self-disciplined and cooperative in line with civic responsibility. In so doing they subscribe to the image of a positive Chinese community acting as a collectivity and in the interest of the general society as an antidote to the negative image blaming China and the Chinese as the source of the coronavirus (Reny and Barreto 2020; S. Wang et al. 2020) especially at the early stage of the pandemic. Within the context of this narrative informal mutual supervision was implemented to monitor whether individual Chinese immigrants in Antwerp were following preventive measures such as two weeks self-quarantine after returning from their Spring Festival visits to China in February 2020, long before the official recommendation of self-quarantine to travelers. Those who were suspected of not respecting the measures were publicly critized on Chinese social media community discussions. It created a sense of peer pressure leading to more self-disciplinary behavior as well as ardent discussions and arguments during the early stage of the pandemic. Some voluntarily limited physical social contact such as refraining from visiting friends and families, canceling travel plans, always wearing highly protective masks, implementing strictive hygiene measures or implementing self-quarantine. This interviewee recalled how some Belgian Chinese immigrants including themselves tried to limit their social contact during the pandemic:

> Chinese in Belgium have taken the pandemic seriously from the beginning. Chinese value life over anything else. We learned mainly from China how to take care of ourselves and what to avoid in the pandemic. I am not afraid, but I am very careful. I always wear a mask when I go out. Almost all Belgian Chinese wear a mask. I don't visit anyone except for my sister, and this is not often. I didn't travel this summer.
>
> (Interviewee 9)

It is also worth noticing that some interviewees recalled and reprimanded family members or friends for not being sufficiently cautious of social contact with non-family members while continuing to meet with their own family members.

Aside from the collective approach to the pandemic, some Belgian Chinese immigrants were also extending acts of solidarity beyond the ethnic boundary. Despite their anxiety on local public's suspicious response to the pandemic, some interviewees tried to offer their protective equipment as a way of taking care of local community. One voluntarily offered one third of her masks and disposable gloves – purchased and posted from China – to her neighbors in the same apartment building. These acts of solidarity were sometimes highly appreciated and reciprocated with gratitude while in other cases, masks were taken but disposable gloves rejected. When the husband of one interviewee offered free medical masks to nearby supermarket staff members, he was met with indifference. Donating protective gear in the pandemic was meant to "protect as many as possible" as interviewee 2 noted, despite the general anti-Chinese climate and the concomitant fear and distress on the part of the Chinese (Reny and Barreto 2020). Another interviewee anonymously donated her only box of masks to the local hospital when she read the news about shortage of personal protective equipment among medical staff. This act gave her sense of self-worth, making her feel like a "full" member of the local community. Similarly, during the early stage of the pandemic in Belgium, some restaurant business owners and various Belgian Chinese immigrant social organizations donated food and anti-epidemic materials to local hospitals and family doctors. These actions have remained under the radar of the mainstream media as they were mainly reported by and within the Chinese immigrant's community although some contact persons from hospitals posted their appreciations on social media. Local mainstream media, such as *Knack*, only covered the two million facemasks donation to Europe from Jack Ma on March 2020.

It is in this context that the CHS was noted by all interviewees as a positive example of how Belgian Chinese immigrants would and have been responding to the pandemic learning from China's approach while adapting to the local context.

Chinese heritage school: localizing "Chinese bubble" in the "Belgium bubble"

The Chinese heritage school in Antwerp was the first Chinese community school in Belgium. It was established in 1994 with the aim to provide Cantonese and Mandarin language and culture classes to pupils of Chinese origin on Wednesday afternoons and Saturdays in Antwerp. Over the course of more than two decades, it has become the largest of 13 Chinese heritage schools in Belgium in terms of student population. Before the pandemic the school had a total number of more than 270 registered students from mostly Chinese origin. Due to its large number of students, the school has ten voluntary Chinese teachers, who are all female Chinese migrants living in Belgium. Over the years, the school, as Chinese community schools elsewhere, has played a role in language education, identity construction and negotiations. More importantly it has become a space for intercultural engagement (Ganassin 2020) for the students, as well as for the female teachers in migratory contexts. When confronted with a global pandemic, the CHS functions as a site of experimentation where Chinese migrants could actively engage in the host and home society while mediating different approaches in coping with the pandemic. In so doing they bridge the "Belgium bubble" and the "Chinese bubble".

The interviewees spoke highly of the CHS's response to the pandemic. They listed three main approaches as highly responsive and effective to the pandemic. Firstly, sanitation measures were timely implemented. CHS temporarily discontinued two weeks of classes in February 2020 to allow those who traveled back from China to have sufficient time to quarantine. It also requested and provided hand gel application at the entrance and in the classroom. Temperature control was mandatory for all those who entered the school, both students and teachers. It limited the amount of people who could enter the school. Mandatory mask wearing (except for students younger than ten) was requested in the classroom from March 2020. Secondly, it offered protective equipment to the teachers and students. To prevent possible exposure to the virus, CHS constantly provided face masks to the teachers.[6] In total, each teacher received at least 100 masks before the second lockdown. Thirdly, it organized timely, well-prepared and high-quality online classes, especially compared to local schools. Despite challenges and pressure to manage ICT skills in only a few weeks and present online language classes, interviewees appreciated the transfer to online education and the opportunity to upgrade their skills. The following interviewee recalled her experience:

> (Switch to) online teaching is a big challenge for me. I have to spend a lot of time to update my skills and practice. But I enjoyed it a lot to exchange with and learn from the colleagues. It's an importance place not only to learn the Chinese language, but also Chinese culture. It's where our culture continues.
>
> (Interviewee 3)

In the trial and error process, the CHS managed to create a new mode of working that contributes to the well-being of the involved players and sense of achievement and continuity (Z. Wang 2020). CHS's responses to the pandemic has been represented by the interviewees as a good example representing Chinese approach to the pandemic in Belgian context where cross-cultural knowledge and coping strategies of Chinese immigrants could be experimented in the host society (Guo et al. 2020).

> CHS is a case in point of Chinese (migrants) protecting ourselves. It indicates a Chinese approach to the pandemic. Fewer students register (at Chinese school). This means Chinese parents distrust in government's measures, thus they'd rather postpone (Chinese learning) for a year. Chinese families prioritize the safety of children because children are our hope, the continuity of our life and culture. The measures taken by CHS reflects Chinese community's approach toward the pandemic.
>
> (Interviewee 10)

CHS is a site where the Chinese migrant community was able to experiment with alternative responses and approaches when being confronted with the pandemic. They assume these experiments to be more effective and protective in the Belgian context. Thus, CHS is the place where the "Belgian bubble" becomes entangled with the "Chinese bubble".

Discussion and conclusion

Trust is fundamental to understanding the impact of the current COVID-19 crisis on different groups and countries across the world at multiscale levels. It is shaping and is shaped by various factors in complex ways. Understanding the dynamics of trust in the context of the current pandemic and migration provides some insights into both the studies of trust and the research of migration. Empirically, we have examined Belgian Chinese migrants' strategies in coping with the pandemic, enquired about their experiences and actions concerning trust during pandemic while living between two worlds, namely their host country and their home country. As this chapter is based on small-scale qualitative research, it doesn't aim to be representative but rather indicative and requires further research on the role of migrant communities and their trust in the host and home societies in the time of crisis. However, we believe the case study of the Chinese migrants' strategies can contribute to our understanding of trust beyond binary choice. In many ways, our findings are largely consistent with the existing trust literature in that trust is related to greater compliance with policy measures. In the context of migrants living in host society, particularly Chinese migrants living in Belgium, they are living in and with two worlds – their home country and their host country. They gain two different perspectives on the pandemic. We have learned from this study that Chinese migrants' trust in the host country is positively associated with received delivery record from related institutions (pragmatical trust) and is negatively related to later adoption of restrictive measures, such as mandatory mask wearing and lockdown policy (positivist trust), political leaders' poor governance, citizens' incompliance with lockdown measures and unpreparedness and low capacity of online education. However, although they appreciate and admire China's effective and restrictive approaches toward the pandemic, they also reflect considerably on the national context of the host country including that of the multiscale political system, geographical locations, size of the country and medical capacities. As a result, the application of similar restrictive measures as in China is considered implausible. Instead, Chinese migrants in Belgium localized what they have learned from China's approaches to the pandemic in a Belgian context. This is what we framed as the localization of "Chinese bubble" in the "Belgian bubble". We learned that migrants' trust should be conceived beyond the binary choice between their host or home country. Migrants, both at individual and collective levels, have the capacity to learn from their home country and adapt these lessons in their host country to create and implement mixed strategies to survive in the time of COVID-19. The acknowledgment of migrants' agency allows for moving beyond the academic debate on the migrants' dichotomy of insider/

outsider or negative connotation and framing of "ethnic enclaves". What is more, it might inform governments across the world to adopt open and inclusive policies toward migrants' ingenuous experiments to counter xenophobia toward immigrant communities in the current responses to the COVID-19 crisis and future recovery (Guadago 2020).

Notes

1 One author was involved with the study site from its establishment in 1994, therefore has a profound knowledge about the history of the site. The other author has been involved with the study site since 2014 and has therefore also established good connections in the field.
2 There are in total 13 Chinese schools in Belgium that are established by Chinese immigrants living in different cities. More than 90% of the voluntary teachers in these schools are female immigrants living in Belgium. We acknowledge possible gender impact on the study. However, this is beyond the scope of this article and can be discussed elsewhere.
3 It took Belgium 653 days to form the current coalition federal government since last election in May 2019 due to its particular system that can make political negotiations difficult to reach an agreement.
4 The interviewee referred to the former federal health minister of Belgium, Maggie de Block, who has been widely criticized for her mismanagement of the coronavirus crisis in the early stage of the pandemic outbreak and the destroy of overdue stocks of personal protective equipment in Belgium.
5 Chinese Embassy in Belgium. February 1, 2020. "Statement on latest information concerning Wuhan Visiting Performers to Belgium" (in Chinese).
6 The CHS received donation of face masks from the Chinese embassy, mainland China, local Chinese associations and Chinese individuals therefore have offered masks to the teachers and its registered students.

References

Abascal, Maria, and Delia Baldassarri. 2015. "Love Thy Neighbor? Ethnoracial Diversity and Trust Reexamined." *American Journal of Sociology* 121 (3): 622–782. https://doi.org/10.1086/683144.

Arfaat, Mohammed. 2020. "Rohingya Efugees Need a Coronavirus Lifeline, Not an Internet Ban." *The New Humanit*. March 24, 2020. https://www.thenewhumanitarian.org/opinion/first-person/2020/03/24/coronavirus-rohingya-refugees-internet-ban-misinformation.

Arrow, Kenneth J. 1972. "Gifts and Exchanges." *Philosophy & Public Affairs* 1 (4): 343–62.

Bachmann, Reinhard. 2011. "At the Crossroads: Future Directions in Trust Research." *Journal of Trust Research* 1 (2): 203–13. https://doi.org/10.1080/21515581.2011.603513.

Balog-Way, Dominic H.P., and Katherine A. McComas. 2020. "COVID-19: Reflections on Trust, Tradeoffs, and Preparedness." *Journal of Risk Research* 23 (7–8): 1–11. https://doi.org/10.1080/13669877.2020.1758192.

Bauer, Paul C. 2015. "Negative Experiences and Trust: A Causal Analysis of the Effects of Victimization on Generalized Trust." *European Sociological Review* 31 (4): 397–417. https://doi.org/10.1093/esr/jcu096.

Bilodeau, Antoine, and Stephen White. 2016. "Trust among Recent Immigrants in Canada: Levels, Roots and Implications for Immigrant Integration." *Journal of Ethnic and Migration Studies* 42 (8): 1317–33. https://doi.org/10.1080/1369183X.2015.1093411.

Coleman, James S. 1988. "Social Capital in the Creation of Human Capital." *Knowledge and Social Capital* 94: 17–42. https://doi.org/10.1086/228943.

Delhey, Jan, Kenneth Newton, and Christian Welzel. 2011. "How General Is Trust in "Most People"? Solving the Radius of Trust Problem." *American Sociological Review* 76 (5): 786–807. https://doi.org/10.1177/0003122411420817.

Devine, Daniel, Jennifer Gaskell, Will Jennings, and Gerry Stoker. 2020. "Trust and the Coronavirus Pandemic: What Are the Consequences of and for Trust? An Early Review of the Literature." *Political Studies Review*, 1–12. https://doi.org/10.1177/1478929920948684.

Dietz, Graham. 2011. "Going Back to the Source: Why Do People Trust Each Other?" *Journal of Trust Research* 1 (2): 215–22. https://doi.org/10.1080/21515581.2011.603514.

Dijck, José van, and Donya Alinead. 2020. "Social Media and Trust in Scientific Expertise: Debating the Covid-19 Pandemic in The Netherlands." *Social Media and Society* 6 (4):1–11. https://doi.org/10.1177/2056305120981057.

Dinesen, Peter Thisted. 2012a. "Does Generalized (Dis)Trust Travel? Examining the Impact of Cultural Heritage and Destination-Country Environment on Trust of Immigrants." *Political Psychology* 33 (4): 495–511. https://doi.org/10.1111/j.1467-9221.2012.00886.x.

———. 2012b. "Parental Transmission of Trust or Perceptions of Institutional Fairness: Generalized Trust of Non-Western Immigrants in a High-Trust Society." *Comparative Politics* 44 (3): 273–89. https://doi.org/10.5129/001041512800078986.

———. 2013. "Where You Come from or Where You Live? Examining the Cultural and Institutional Explanation of Generalized Trust Using Migration as a Natural Experiment." *European Sociological Review* 29 (1): 114–28. https://doi.org/10.1093/esr/jcr044.

Dinesen, Peter Thisted, and Marc Hooghe. 2010. "When in Rome, Do as the Romans Do: The Acculturation of Generalized Trust among Immigrants in Western Europe." *International Migration Review* 44 (3): 697–727. https://doi.org/10.1111/j.1747-7379.2010.00822.x.

Dinesen, Peter Thisted, and Kim Mannemar Sønderskov. 2018. "Ethnic Diversity and Social Trust." In *The Oxford Handbook of Social and Political Trust*, edited by Eric Uslaner, 175–204. Oxford: Oxford University Press.

———. 2015. "Ethnic Diversity and Social Trust: Evidence from the Micro-Context." *American Sociological Review* 80 (3): 550–73. https://doi.org/10.1177/0003122415577989.

Doerr, Neriko Musha, and Kiri Lee. 2009. "Contesting Heritage: Language, Legitimacy, and Schooling at a Weekend Japanese-Language School in the United States." *Language and Education* 23 (5): 425–41. https://doi.org/10.1080/09500780802651706.

Durkheim, Emile. 1984. *The Division of Labor in Society. Zeitschrift Für Sozialforschung*. Vol. 3. The Macmillan Press Ltd. https://doi.org/10.5840/zfs19343310.

Evans, John H., and Eszter Hargittai. 2020. "Who Doesn't Trust Fauci? The Public's Belief in the Expertise and Shared Values of Scientists in the COVID-19 Pandemic." *Socius: Sociological Research for a Dynamic World* 6: 237802312094733. https://doi.org/10.1177/2378023120947337.

Fukuyama, Francis. 1995. *Trust: The Social Virtues and the Creation of Prosperity*. New York: Free Press. http://www.bravo-mag.com/25-nigerian-ceos-in-fraud-scandal/.

Ganassin, Sara. 2020. *Language, Culture and Identity in Two Chinese Community Schools. More than One Way of Being Chinese?* Bristol: Multilingual Matters.

Gao, Zhipeng. 2021. "Unsettled Belongings: Chinese Immigrants' Mental Health Vulnerability as a Symptom of International Politics in the COVID-19 Pandemic." *Journal of Humanistic Psychology* 61 (2): 198–218.

Glanville J.L., Paxton P. 2007. "How Do We Learn to Trust ? A Confirmatory Tetrad Analysis of the Sources of Generalized Trust Author (s): Jennifer L. Glanville and Pamela Paxton How Do We Learn to Trust ? Fi Confirmatory Tetrad Analysis of the Sources of Generalized Trust *." *Social Psychology Quarterly* 70 (3): 230–42.

Greenaway, Christina, Sally Hargreaves, Sapha Barkati, Christina M. Coyle, Federico Gobbi, Apostolos Veizis, and Paul Douglas. 2020. "COVID-19: Exposing and Addressing Health Disparities among Ethnic Minorities and Migrants." *Journal of Travel Medicine* 27 (7): 1–3. https://doi.org/10.1093/jtm/taaa113.

Guadago, Lorenzo. 2020. *Migrants and the COVID-19 Pandemic : An Initial Analysis*. Geneva. Lorenzo: International Organization for Migration.

Guo, Mengna, Mar Joanpere, Cristina Pulido, and Maria Padrós Cuxart. 2020. "Coping of Chinese Citizens Living in Spain during the COVID-19 Pandemic: Lessons for Personal Well-Being and Social Cohesion." *Sustainability* 12 (19). https://doi.org/10.3390/SU12197949.

Habermas, Jürgen, and Transl. by Shierry W. Nicholsen and Jerry A. Stark. 1988. *On the Logic of the Social Sciences*. Cambridge, MA: The MIT Press.

Hardin, Russell. 2002. *Trust and Trustworthiness*. New York: Russell Sage Foundation.

Helliwell, John F., Shun Wang, and Jinwen Xu. 2016. "How Durable Are Social Norms? Immigrant Trust and Generosity in 132 Countries." *Social Indicators Research* 128 (1): 201–19. https://doi.org/10.1007/s11205-015-1026-2.

Hsu, Hsiu-Pei, Ching Lin Pang, and Wim Haagdorens. 2012. "Writing as Cultural Practice: Case Study of a Chinese Heritage School in Belgium." *Procedia: Social and Behavioral Sciences* 47: 1592–96. https://doi.org/10.1016/j.sbspro.2012.06.868.

Isaeva, Neve, Reinhard Bachmann, Alexandra Bristow, and Mark N.K. Saunders. 2015. "Why the Epistemologies of Trust Researchers Matter." *Journal of Trust Research* 5 (2): 153–69. https://doi.org/10.1080/21515581.2015.1074585.

Kim, Jinhee. 2011. "Korean Immigrant Mothers' Perspectives: The Meanings of a Korean Heritage Language School for Their Children's American Early Schooling Experiences." *Early Childhood Education Journal* 39 (2): 133–41. https://doi.org/10.1007/s10643-011-0453-1.

Kinnvall, Catarina. 2016. "The Postcolonial Has Moved into Europe: Bordering, Security and Ethno-Cultural Belonging." *Journal of Common Market Studies* 54 (1): 152–68. https://doi.org/10.1111/jcms.12326.

Krause, Elizabeth L., and Massimo Bressan. 2020. "Viral Encounters: Xenophobia, Solidarity, and Place-Based Lessons from Chinese Migrants in Italy." *Human Organization* 79 (4): 259–70.

Kye, Bongoh, and Sun Jae Hwang. 2020. "Social Trust in the Midst of Pandemic Crisis: Implications from COVID-19 of South Korea." *Research in Social Stratification and Mobility* 68 (June): 100523. https://doi.org/10.1016/j.rssm.2020.100523.

Liu, Wei, Xiao Guang Yue, and Paul B. Tchounwou. 2020. "Response to the Covid-19 Epidemic: The Chinese Experience and Implications for Other Countries." *International*

Journal of Environmental Research and Public Health 17 (7): 1–6. https://doi.org/10.3390/IJERPH17072304.

Ljunge, Martin. 2014. "Trust Issues: Evidence on the Intergenerational Trust Transmission among Children of Immigrants." *Journal of Economic Behavior and Organization* 106 (2012): 175–96. https://doi.org/10.1016/j.jebo.2014.07.001.

Longstaff, P H, and Sung-Un Yang. 2008. "Communication Management and Trust: Their Role in Building Resilience to "Surprises" Such as Natural Disasters, Pandemic Flu, and Terrorism." *Ecology and Society* 13 (1): 3. http://digitalcommons.usu.edu/unf_research%0Ahttp://www.ecologyandsociety.org/vol13/iss1/art3/.

Lovari, Alessandro. 2020. "Spreading (Dis)Trust: Covid-19 Misinformation and Government Intervention in Italy." *Media and Communication* 8 (2): 458–61. https://doi.org/10.17645/mac.v8i2.3219.

Luhmann, Niklas. 1979. *Trust and Power*. New York: John Wiley & Sons.

Ma, Yingyi, and Ning Zhan. 2020. "To Mask or Not to Mask amid the COVID-19 Pandemic: How Chinese Students in America Experience and Cope with Stigma." *Chinese Sociological Review* 54 (1): 1–26. https://doi.org/10.1080/21620555.2020.1833712.

Moschion, Julie, and Domenico Tabasso. 2014. "Trust of Second-Generation Immigrants: Intergenerational Transmission or Cultural Assimilation?" *IZA Journal of Migration* 3 (1): 1–30. https://doi.org/10.1186/2193-9039-3-10.

Nannestad, Peter, Gert Tinggaard Svendsen, Peter Thisted Dinesen, and Kim Mannemar Sønderskov. 2014. "Do Institutions or Culture Determine the Level of Social Trust? The Natural Experiment of Migration from Non-Western to Western Countries." *Journal of Ethnic and Migration Studies* 40 (4): 544–65. https://doi.org/10.1080/1369183X.2013.830499.

Parsons, Talcott. n.d. *The Structure of Social Actions*. New York: Free Press.

Paxton, Pamela. 2007. "Association Memberships and Generalized Trust: A Multilevel Model across 31 Countries." *Social Forces* 86 (1): 47–76. https://doi.org/10.1353/sof.2007.0107.

Paxton, Pamela, and Jennifer L. Glanville. 2015. "Is Trust Rigid or Malleable? A Laboratory Experiment." *Social Psychology Quarterly* 78 (2): 194–204. https://doi.org/10.1177/0190272515582177.

Reny, Tyler T., and Matt A. Barreto. 2020. "Xenophobia in the Time of Pandemic: Othering, Anti-Asian Attitudes, and COVID-19." *Politics, Groups, and Identities* 10 (2): 1–24. https://doi.org/10.1080/21565503.2020.1769693.

Rice, Tom W., and Jan L. Feldman. 1997. "Civic Culture and Democracy from Europe to America." *Journal of Politics* 59 (4): 1143–72. https://doi.org/10.2307/2998596.

Roberts, Hannah. 2020. "How Italy's "Little China" Dodged the Coronavirus." *POLITICO* 2020. https://www.politico.eu/article/how-italys-little-china-dodged-the-coronavirus/.

Rothstein, Bo, and Eric M. Uslaner. 2005. "All for All: Equality, Corruption, and Social Trust." *World Politics* 58 (1): 41–72. https://doi.org/10.1353/wp.2006.0022.

Simmel, Georg. 2004. *The Philosophy of Money. The Philosophy of Money*. Third edition. London and New York: Routledge. https://doi.org/10.4324/9780203828298.

Simpson, Brent, Tucker McGrimmon, and Kyle Irwin. 2007. "Are Blacks Really Less Trusting than Whites? Revisiting the Race and Trust Question." *Social Forces* 86 (2): 525–52. https://doi.org/10.1093/sf/86.2.525.

Soroka, Stuart, Richard Johnston, and Keith Banting. 2007. "Ethnicity, Trust, and the Welfare State." In *Diversity, Social Capital and the Welfare State*, edited by Fiona

Kay and Richard Johnston, 279–303. Vancouver, BC: University of British Columbia Press.

Tillmar, Malin. 2012. "Cross-Cultural Comparative Case Studies: A Means of Uncovering Dimensions of Trust." In *Handbook of Research Methods on Trust*, edited by Fergus Lyon, Guido Möllering, and Mark N.K. Saunders, 102–9. Cheltenham: Edward Elgar Publishing Limited. https://doi.org/10.4337/9780857932013.

Uslaner, Eric M. 2008. "Where You Stand Depends upon Where Your Grandparents Sat: The Inheritability of Generalized Trust." *Public Opinion Quarterly* 72 (4): 725–40. https://doi.org/10.1093/poq/nfn058.

Wang, Simeng, Xiabing Chen, Yong Li, Chloé Luu, Ran Yan, and Francesco Madrisotti. 2020. ""I'm More Afraid of Racism than of the Virus!": Racism Awareness and Resistance among Chinese Migrants and Their Descendants in France during the Covid-19 Pandemic." *European Societies* 23 (1): S721–42. https://doi.org/10.1080/14616696.2020.1836384.

Wang, Zi. 2020. "Addressing Migrants' Well-Being during COVID-19: An Analysis of Chinese Communities' Heritage Language Schools in Germany." *Migration Studies* 9 (3): 1144–65. https://doi.org/10.1093/migration/mnaa033.

Wong, Catherine Mei Ling, and Olivia Jensen. 2020. "The Paradox of Trust: Perceived Risk and Public Compliance during the COVID-19 Pandemic in Singapore." *Journal of Risk Research* 23 (7–8): 1021–30. https://doi.org/10.1080/13669877.2020.1756386.

Wu, Cary. 2020. "Does Migration Affect Trust? Internal Migration and the Stability of Trust among Americans." *Sociological Quarterly* 61 (3): 523–43. https://doi.org/10.1080/00380253.2019.1711259.

Wu, Cary, and Rima Wilkes. 2016. "Durable Power and Generalized Trust in Everyday Social Exchange." *Proceedings of the National Academy of Sciences of the United States of America* 113 (11): E1417. https://doi.org/10.1073/pnas.1523536113.

Yoon, Myeong Sook, Israel Fisseha Feyissa, and So-Won Suk. 2021. "Panic and Trust during COVID-19: A Cross-Sectional Study on Immigrants in South Korea." *Healthcare* 9 (2): 199. https://doi.org/10.3390/healthcare9020199.

9 "Fear not the want of armor, for mine is also yours to wear"

Trust and community cultivation for risk response of a Chinese immigrant group in the United States

Qiaoyun Zhang and Ziying You[1]

Introduction

This chapter explores why and how a Chinese immigrant group in the American state of Florida engaged in the donation of face masks to local public service institutions amidst the COVID-19 pandemic. The Chinese immigrant group's management of the face masks, including the acknowledgment, use, purchase and donation of them, was their first and foremost response to the COVID-19 pandemic after its outbreak in late February of 2020. Interestingly, the Chinese volunteer group was organized under the leadership of the local Chinese language school – Huagen Chinese School – where the majority of the participants were also leaders, teachers, student-parents and volunteers at the school. Analyzing Huagen as a characteristic social center of the particular Chinese immigrant group of the city of Gainesville in Florida, this chapter argues that the Chinese immigrant group's face mask donation relied on the co-constitutive process of trust building and community cultivation strategies within the local society. Specifically, the chapter reveals the community-based enactment of trust in promoting organized group actions in times of risk situations.

Given the contingent and precarious nature of the COVID-19 pandemic, the inter- and intra-community trust that enabled the donation of face masks across American and Chinese societies was generated "in unpredictable forms extraneous to social solidarity, exchange networks, or kinship" (Rubaii 2020, 212). As Rubaii (ibid., 212) argues, trust in the crisis context becomes enunciatory. This term is borrowed from anthropologist Kim Fortun (2001) who, in her research on the advocacy after the Bhopal disaster in India, describes how parties of divergent yet irreconcilable interests – including doctors, lawyers, corporate executives and environmental justice activists – in the United States formed a fleeting group to deal with the aftermath of the incident. In Rubaii's (2020, 212) study on the medication smuggling network in ISIS-controlled northern Iraq, he uses the enunciatory trust to illustrate the articulation, function and affection of the contingent trust network "traversing divergent interests".

The Huagen case further provokes us to investigate the roots and impacts of the enunciatory trust in the host community. Following Lim's argument (in this

DOI: 10.4324/9781003291220-9

volume), the chapter analyzes the social trust during and after the trust liminality, to reveal the cultivation of trust through consistent socio-historical and cultural-political practice long before the actual risk takes place (Jimenez 2011). A global risk threat such as the coronavirus oftentimes leads to a crisis of science and governance. This is because unknown and "liminal" risks like the COVID-19 can render established knowledge and authorities especially vulnerable and suspicious. It is even more difficult to advocate for the unprecedented and sometimes uninviting information and policies when the public lacked the familiar experiences or cultural knowledge to comprehend them.

We propose that moral responsibilities and affective attachment brought out by a trustful relationship are essential for people's risk perception and responses. Particular knowledge making, identity building and affective strategies are cornerstones of establishing and maintaining a trustful relationship and, in turn, promoting collective community risk response. The making of a strong, compassionate and impactful Chinese immigrant community demonstrates the changing identity, values and capability of the highly educated Chinese students and professionals immigrating to the United States since the establishment of China's Open Door Policy. The Chinese desire for and devotion to engaging in community affairs allowed them to become active volunteers during the COVID-19 pandemic.

In the following sections, the chapter first explains the development of Huagen Chinese Language School as a representative collective of the Chinese immigrants in Gainesville and analyzes the characteristics leading to the group's engagement with the local community. It then closely studies the face mask donation process to reveal the characteristics of emergency formation of trust relationships. The chapter continues to examine how the Chinese immigrant group, gaining support from the face mask donation activity, can further develop a trusting relationship to override crises of science and racial identity during COVID-19. The process has not only shaped the immigrant group's relationship with the local community, but also negotiated their marginalized identity while fighting against distrust and discrimination from people in both the US and China.

The chapter draws on structured interviews about the purchase, use and donation of face masks among leaders and active members of Huagen Chinese Language School. As one of the researchers lived in Gainesville throughout the donation period, we were able to witness and participate in the initiative, as well as befriend and interview the key players between March and June 2020. The study is part of a research project which investigates Chinese people's experience of and adaptation to the COVID-19 pandemic in the US. More than 50 interviews and counting have been conducted since the pandemic's outbreak. The project is supported by research projects on cultural adaptation to contemporary risk initiated by researchers in China and the US.[2] The structured interviews adopted the method of life storytelling which asked the interviewees to fully introduce their life experiences before discussing the face mask donation. Discourse analysis methods were used to tease out the main themes and common concerns of all interviews.

Community rootedness of Huagen

The Huagen Chinese Language School is located in the city of Gainesville, Florida. In Chinese, Huagen means "Chinese roots", a name that clearly indicates the school's mission of transmitting and disseminating the Chinese language and culture within the local Chinese community and beyond. The Chinese language school was established in 1997 by a small group of Mandarin-speaking parents, most of whom emigrated to the United States (US) from mainland China. The parents were concerned about their American-born children's Chinese language learning environment. The school started with a few Chinese classes offered at home and taught by the concerned parents with self-made textbooks. Given their sociopolitical upbringing, they taught Mandarin Chinese, the official language used in mainland China. As more parents and students joined the classes, the school developed into one of the biggest local Chinese language schools with more than 100 students. The school was officially certified as a non-profit organization (NPO) in the early 2000s.

Huagen's development into an influential fully fledged Chinese language and culture teaching and sharing center reflected the changing composition and sociality of the Mandarin-speaking population in Gainesville and, to a large extent, that of the Mandarin-speaking immigrants to the US since the late 1970s. These migrants went to the US at a time when China arguably transformed into a post-socialist state and allowed its members more opportunities to explore the world. The changes can be summarized in the following three ways.

First, Gainesville, along with the rest of the US, has witnessed a large influx of educated young students and professionals originally from mainland China following the initiation of China's Open Door Policy in the late 1970s. Since the late 19th century, Florida has seen surges of Chinese immigrants (Mohl 1995). Similar to that in other American states, early Chinese immigrants mainly engaged in manual labor and small business (e.g., laundry businesses, truck farms and grocery stores) in Florida (ibid., 264–265). After the initiation of the Immigrant Act of 1965, Asians became the fastest-growing foreign-born group in Florida (ibid., 262). Such a trend has continued in the 21st century (Rayer 2017). In Alachua County where the University of Florida (UF) is located, the Asian population increased nine-fold between 1970 and 1990. In the immigration surge, Chinese and Indians were the two major groups. A survey published in 2017 revealed that 12% of the foreign-born individuals in Gainesville were born in China (ibid.).

More importantly, a different immigrant group has arrived there. Since the 1970s, the majority of the new Asian immigrants have been the "professors, students, and medical personnel at the university's medical school and large teaching hospital" (Mohl 1995, 280). The recent data published by the University of Florida's international office showed that the 2,253 Chinese students were by far the largest foreign student body on campus. According to our interview data, a good number of the PhD students, especially medical doctors, have chosen to stay and work at the university-affiliated hospital and the associated laboratories after graduation. Some have moved to Gainesville after getting their higher degrees in other states to work at the University of Florida and its associated research and health institutions.

Secondly, the educated Chinese immigrant group in Gainesville has different ways to maintain and transmit the Chinese language and culture. Floridian Chinese communities have long traditions of keeping and promoting their cultural roots (Mohl 1995). Traditionally, Chinese languages and cultures were taught, displayed and maintained through teaching Chinese languages (previously, this was mainly Cantonese and Taiwanese) and organizing ritual activities in different immigrant enclaves across the state of Florida. In Gainesville, Chinese culture and traditions have been mainly transmitted at Chinese language schools, probably because of the large number of educated professionals. Among the three Chinese language schools that exist there, Huagen is quite special. It was founded by then UF student-parents from mainland China and has been teaching Mandarin Chinese in simplified Chinese since the very beginning. The other two Chinese language schools founded by immigrants from Hong Kong and Taiwan offered Cantonese courses and Taiwanese in complicated traditional Chinese, respectively. According to our informants, Huagen started by teaching Mandarin Chinese because that was the language spoken and written by the founding teacher-parents there. For years it has continued with this teaching design, and purposely chosen textbooks of the proper formats. In this case, Huagen has represented the cultural and identity preferences of the new Chinese immigrant group – highly educated students and professionals from mainland China – in Gainesville.

Thirdly, an analysis of Huagen's teaching and extra-curriculum activities reveals that Huagen has long aimed to be a Chinese cultural transmission and activity center for not only children of the immigrants, but also all community members. Huagen's Chinese courses are open to all interested young children. A few years ago, it started the free "Happy Chinese" program for children and adults from non-Mandarin-speaking families or with no Chinese language immersion. According to the president of Huagen, the Happy Chinese program aimed to allow more community members to utilize the school's services and meet the Mandarin-speaking folks. As Huagen grew in scale more volunteers including both Chinese and American parents and friends joined in and initiated several non-language activities for both the students, parents and others. For example, an American volunteer who was once a local champion taught Huagen's chess class. With his leadership, students already won several regional titles. One of the students, Tianhui (Cindy) Jie, qualified to be on the US delegation to the World Youth Chess Championships in 2014. The soccer coach, also an American volunteer, led Huagen's team, composed of students of different racial backgrounds, into the semi-final game of the local students' soccer tournament. There were traditional arts and arts courses for parents and other adult members. Gradually, Huagen has grown its roots in the local community by providing inexpensive language, cultural, arts and sports activities for all interested members. Since all members of Huagen work there as volunteers, it only charges reasonably priced tuition to cover its rent and other essential expenses.

In addition, Huagen has been paying great attention to developing its connection with the local community in various ways. More than merely attracting people to its courses, it has organized annual fundraising events and community service activities so as to reach out to the Gainesville neighborhoods. Traditionally, Chinese immigrant organizations and language schools would organize events such as the Chinese Spring Festival Gala and Chinese composition competitions catering to the interests of the immigrant groups. According to Mohl's (1995) research on such organizations in Florida during the late 20th century, the organizations might not intend to either invite the non-Chinese community members to participate or make the events part of the community experience. Huagen, however, sought to become a local institution from the very beginning.

The most noticeable event is the annual Joey's Run & Food Fest co-hosted by Huagen and the NPO, Joey's Wings, in honor of Joey Xu, a Gainesville native and former Huagen student who died of a rare kidney cancer in 2014. Aiming to advocate for the research and treatment of kidney cancers in young children, Joey's Wings started the annual fundraising event in Gainesville with the support of Huagen in 2015, which attracted participants beyond the Huagen's members. Recently, Huagen and Joey's Wings co-sponsored other projects such as the Zumba fundraiser program to help families with kidney cancer patients.

Joey's Wings, together with Huagen, represented a new kind of NPOs established by Chinese immigrants. As research promotion and teaching organizations, respectively, Joey's Wings and Huagen purposely engaged in advocating for advanced knowledge and community mutual help throughout their programs. Such endeavors were made possible because of the high education levels of the founders and participants, reflecting the changing composition of the Chinese immigrants in Gainesville. The success of such organizations demonstrated the immigrant group's capacity of engaging in and influencing American medical, legislative and educational resources. For example, founders of the Joey's Wings lobbied for the passing of the congressional act for childhood cancer and advocated for the application of the latest cancer treatment on young children in select hospitals nationwide.

Briefly tracing the history and achievements of Huagen, we have tried to examine the main characteristics of the local Chinese immigrant group composing of educated students, professors and professionals mostly from mainland China. They have had and maintained close connections with their Chinese family members and friends. The majority finished high school and college education in China before going to the US for higher education. Some of them had years of work experience in China before they left. With the establishment and development of Huagen, they have expended great efforts in developing their roots in the local community with their expertise and compassion. The new Chinese immigrants have demonstrated strong desire to nurture trust and respectability in an American community through engaging with local affairs, advocating for advanced knowledge and mutual help, as well as promoting Chinese languages and cultures.

Through long-term community trust-building efforts the Chinese immigrants established their community identity and belonging. The Chinese immigrants' capacity and desire to gain trust and support from the local community reflects their changed identity politics and socioeconomic power. They are representatives of the international Chinese, who are eager to take the best of the cultures they encounter to enhance their positive and public identity as concerned citizens. It was their deep connectedness with both their country of origin – mainland China – and new homes – Gainesville – that empowered them with the willingness, capacity and influence in the face mask donation during the COVID-19 pandemic.

Face mask donations during the COVID-19 outbreak

Gainesville's Chinese immigrants were well informed of and greatly concerned with the COVID-19 pandemic long before other groups were, due to the fact that their families and friends in China began fighting a difficult war against the coronavirus in late January, 2020. Huagen Chinese Language School made a quick response. It canceled its 2020 Spring Festival Gala scheduled in early February. Three weeks later, it canceled all its spring courses. With the classes and activities canceled, its participants were left with little to do at the school, but much worry about their own families and close ones at home and in China.

Some members carried on their volunteering spirit. In late February and early March, a small number – about 15 – of concerned members in Gainesville, who were also Huagen's administrators, teachers and student-parents, organized a group to plan for donating face masks to hospitals in Hubei, China, then the most affected Chinese province. Some of the volunteers were also doctors and medical service providers at the local hospital. According to the president of Huagen, the group was formed purely based on volunteerism and later decided that Huagen could be an ideal organization for such efforts:

> People were thinking that since there was no Chinese business association or something [in Gainesville], so then the Chinese school was the best carrier. [To donate face masks] in the name of Chinese schools on the one hand could build up reputation for the school, and on the other hand could do something together for the community, which was also good for community coherence. For example, if you needed to buy something or use a bank account [in the donation], one could borrow the account of the Chinese school. Just from the financial aspect, how to say? [The use of the school account] can be tracked. It's much better than a private account. It's a public account. So that's the story.

It is worth noting at that point in Gainesville, only the Chinese immigrants started to wear face masks outside. They learned this from their friends and family members in mainland China, who had been required to wear face masks in public since the outbreak of the pandemic in late January. There appeared a sharp shortage of face masks in mainland China, which made the overseas groups realize the need for donations. The donation was carried out by individual efforts. According to our interviews with the participants, there was no involvement or incentive from Chinese authorities or associations in the US at this stage of donation. The group of 15 was divided into several task teams to handle the purchase, transportation and actual donation of the face masks. In mid-March, about 100 boxes of the 100-pack face masks were donated to designated hospitals. Until this point, Huagen members and their friends acted as helpers and caring partners to their mother country. The face masks were donated in the names of the Huagen Chinese School and Gainesville Chinese Community. As the first round of donations reached their destination at the desired time, the success encouraged the volunteers to do more as they saw the pandemic situation worsen in the United States.

In late March, the pandemic spread out in the US. As the situation became more and more serious, the US experienced a similar shortage of personal protection equipment (PPE) as China did. Huagen's team members quickly realized the severity of the situation and campaigned for the donation of face masks to local hospitals. According to volunteer D:

> [The news was] from all aspects of the media here, such as on Facebook. Everyone will say this. Not only here [Gainesville], but the United States did not have enough [PPE] ... If doctors and nurses fall down, and if the community members are diagnosed, who will treat them? Finally, it will come to the people in the community. All of us will shoulder the consequences. Therefore, we think that local hospitals and medical institutions should be the first priority. It may be a drop in the bucket to make donations to them. But at least it shows our community's intention and support to the community.

Quickly, the volunteer team formed a larger and more cohesive group when more members of different backgrounds of the Huagen School community and related friends voluntarily joined in. Huagen Chinese Language School was then unofficially named as the leading organization to handle mostly the financial aspects of the donation. The president of the school also became the leader of the face mask donation team that coordinated all activities.

The donation was managed with extensive planning and organization – highlighting the new immigrant group's specific intellectual, economic and social power which allowed them to help their host community. One of the first challenges of the face mask donation was to look for the right PPE to donate to the right places. The other challenge was to ensure the donation was qualified and trustworthy. The controversy of face mask wearing was heightened throughout the pandemic. The donation team was also aware of it. Instead of engaging in ethical or moral arguments, the team resorted to professional knowledge and experience:

> Because there were some people in our planning group. They were Chinese doctors or Chinese nurses in the hospital, and they were also in our planning group. Actually, they had little to do with the Chinese School at that time. Some of their children grew older [and left the school], and some of them might not attend the Chinese School. But when we had discussions in

> the group, we naturally talked about this [what and where to donate]. It was natural [to think that way]. They didn't know very clearly what to do, but after such a chat, everyone knew and thought in that direction.

The team relied on the local institutions' trust and support to accomplish its mission. From the beginning, the team utilized their exclusive information resources and extended communication networks with the UF Health systems in order to decide what and where to donate the face masks. The parents and friends of Huagen, who were also doctors and medical service professionals at the university hospital, provided the donation team with expert and up-to-date information on what the hospital needed. According to our interview with volunteer D:

> Here we have the university hospital of the UF, which is a very large general hospital in Southeast America. This hospital is equivalent to a central hospital in this area, which also serves [patients] such as in Louisiana, Alabama, Florida and North Carolina. Our hospital serves this area, so it is a very large general hospital. The flow of people and the number of patients are very large. At the beginning, we were thinking, if this is the case, as we knew the shortage of medical resources in Wuhan, and if the patient [number] goes up, it is impossible for the local hospital to have enough capacity to cope with such a large-scale infectious disease. So from our point of view, we were thinking about how to first protect our local hospital's medical staff, which meant that we had to prepare enough medical resources for them, including face masks and protective clothing. We wanted to buy these things.

The health professionals provided the donation team with advice about what kinds of face masks and other PPE to purchase, teaching the face mask purchase task group members to distinguish various kinds of medical face masks so as to secure the proper ones for hospital use. According to another volunteer W:

> Some of our four or five volunteers in the team work in the hospital. For example, I used to work in the hospital, but I left in February. I would know the situation in the whole hospital, such as the inventory of the protective devices and the shortage. So we started from this point of view and contacted local [organizations] for donation.

More importantly, the doctors and nurses helped identify the qualified products with proper certificates to increase the credibility of the donation. In March 2020, there was a global shortage of proper PPE and other medical devices for coronavirus treatment. With its quick response to the outbreak and massive factory infrastructure, China soon became the world production center for essential medical devices where many factories and companies crowded in to produce such equipment. Yet the quality of the products produced by the newly transformed factories, some of which were previously diaper or clothing factories, needed to be further examined.

Reports of non-certified PPE being circulated at home and abroad raised global concern of the trustworthiness of the Chinese products. With the help and endorsement of the medical professionals, Huagen's donation team learned to look for products with certifications issued by both the Chinese and American governments. Once the team secured a new face mask producer, they would immediately send the sample face masks to the professionals for further examination. This cross-check procedure greatly reduced the risk of getting the improper products and increased the team's efficiency and credibility.

In the meantime, face mask donation required substantial financing and communication capacities of the donation team to manage the donation in Gainesville as well as purchase and transportation of face masks in mainland China. The donation critically tested Huagen's trustworthiness within the local community. As Huagen already formed a team to carry out the donation procedures, it started a quick campaign for money donations inside the Gainesville Chinese community. However, Huagen's president told us that the campaign was actually not needed since many community members took the initiatives to donate early on. Before the donation campaign started, the team decided to use Huagen Chinese School's bank account as the designated account to receive donations and record expenditures. An accounting team was responsible for recording and announcing to the whole donation group, and on Huagen's school website, every donation and expenditure on the account. The school account's weekly cash flows were made public so that everyone engaged in the activity could supervise it.

The donation team depended upon the Huagen's community reputation to promote its activities, which in turn, enhanced the school and the Chinese community's community engagement and influence. According to volunteer W:

> In this way, if we [the volunteers] launch a large-scale initiative to raise funds, individual people may have doubts. So at that time, we think that we can simply borrow the platform of the Chinese School, because this platform is a non-profit organization … The Chinese School was equivalent to the legal representative of our whole community. Of course, we couldn't represent the whole Chinese community. We couldn't say that as some of the older children in the whole Chinese community might not be in the Chinese school, or some of them had moved to other places. They didn't associate with the Chinese school. But they were still actively involved in the process of service.

When the money was in place, the donation team set out to search for the proper face masks at a time when the PPE was globally in short supply. To secure a large number of qualified face masks exemplified the donation team's bilingual and cross-cultural communication skills and networks, which were also distinct characteristics of the new-generation Chinese immigrants in the US. The team had to make sure that the face masks donated were suitable for hospital use. It was based on the team's frequent and close communication with UF Health's management group. The latter gave the donation team daily updates of the hospital's stock information, while the donation team informed the management group of their capacities. According to several of the volunteers interviewed, the hospital's management trusted their efforts from the beginning.

The trust was also further built up during the crisis situation when the donation team strived to establish itself as an able and trustworthy partner. To reciprocate the hospital's trust, the team took great efforts to ensure the quality and quantity of the donation, which was particularly hard to accomplish. The purchase team was then divided into seven or eight small groups, each group responsible for contacting a specific supplier, checking their products against FDA (Food and Drug Administration) standards, coordinating their contacts in China to examine the samples and compare the prices. All of the tasks required the purchase team to have an extensive and efficient network in China. As volunteer D told:

> Because we knew that the supply of goods was very tight at that time. The policy of domestic customs clearance could change three times a day. In the morning, the contact people in China said that the [face masks] could go through the customs, but by noon, the policy might have changed. So at that time, the purchase contact team was very frustrated … At the same time, you know that we were in the United States. Our contact with China was more through the introduction of friends. We had little idea of the reliability of the factories or the payees. So we needed to avoid being cheated. Because if we lost the money, we could not explain it to the local donors.

When the face masks finally reached Gainesville, the donation team had to carefully organize the actual donation activities. As the face masks were greatly needed across the hospital departments, the team was challenged with balancing the priorities and fairness of the donation. The decision was made not based on personal preferences or connections, but again on scientific and realistic judgment. Although the volunteers revealed to us that there were quarrels among the team members about where the face masks should go, they reached an agreement by consulting informants at the hospital. The first batches of face masks were given to the departments most in need. The donation team placed a special emphasis on public promotion and relationship building throughout the whole donation process. The charitable campaign helped enhance the bonding between the Mandarin-speaking immigrants and their host community. The donation team established a media task group to follow the donation process.

The special efforts of media representation show that the contemporary Chinese immigrant group was very sensitive to image and identity building within the local community, which exemplified the group's urge to integrate with and influence the community lives. To promote and commemorate the generous contribution, volunteers created a poster for the event, which was printed out and pasted on each of the packing boxes of the face masks donated. The poster featured a mask-wearing panda and a gator giving a high-five to each other. The panda represented the Chinese in general, and the gator represented the Gainesville community, and to be more specific, the University of Florida, as the UF football team is nick-named "the Gators". On the top of the poster written in Chinese was "岂曰无衣, 与子同裳", which literally meant "Fear not the want of armor, for mine is also yours to wear". Next to the two mascots written in English was "United We Stand". On the bottom of the poster written in red was "Gainesville Chinese Community PPE DONATION".

When the team donated more than 8,000 face masks and other PPE to the UF Health facilities on April 3, 2020, local news reporters were invited to witness the event and interview the leading organizers. Xiuli Liu, a pathologist at UF Health and donation organizer, said in front of the camera, "just a lot of effort, this is a collective effort from the entire Chinese American community in Gainesville". The news report was then broadcast on the local WCJB-TV channel. *The Gainesville Sun*, the local newspaper, and the *Independent Florida Alligator*, UF's newspaper, published long reports and interviews with the key organizers, respectively. The use of social media sites such as Facebook and Twitter was emphasized. The media task group posted regular updates on such sites to communicate publicly with the concerned audience about the donation process. The reports also attracted many non-Chinese members to participate in the donation.

The whole donation process started in early March and continued until late May, 2020. The donation began at a time when the UF Health's whole system was in desperate need of PPE and ended when the system was able to secure a steady supply of such equipment. The donation supported the Gainesville community until it could stand on its own feet again. In total, it collected close to $40,000 worth of donations and donated more than 20,000 face masks and other PPE to UF Health facilities, Gainesville police offices and other public service institutions. Although the majority of the donations came from the Mandarin-speaking members, some of it was also collected from non-Chinese friends and families who were involved in the campaign from the early start.

Enunciatory trust and community cultivation for risk responses

In the interviews, the volunteers repeatedly emphasized that the trust of the Gainesville community was fundamental for the successful completion of the face mask donation. As volunteer D comments, "If one wants to have a foothold in America, one must be honest and gain trust from others". Such a comment reveals two important factors leading to a successful local community's response to the COVID-19 pandemic. The first defining factor is trust, which can promote collective action in times of unprecedented risk situations. Sociological studies have recognized that trust is a critical means for people to deal with uncertainty (Levi 2015, 664; Levi and Stoker 2000; see also Holton 1994; Jimenez 2011). Yet threats like the COVID-19 pandemic can largely undermine people's risk judgment capacity. Douglas' (1986) investigation of risk acceptance argues that people's risk response is profoundly influenced by cultural perceptions and social resources (see also Douglas and Wildavsky 1983).

As the Huagen case reveals, enunciatory trust established in crisis can be liminal and fleeting. Inside Huagen, the face mask donation task force groups quickly developed and dissolved within three month. The Huagen group's communication and transaction with the Chinese domestic face mask factories stopped after the deliveries of the face masks. Huagen reassumed its role as a Chinese language center in the following fall semester. The interviewers even confessed to us that they did not communicate with each other for a long time after the donation. The trust network becomes effective depending on the emergency of the event. It is "tenuous, dissipate[s] quickly, and at times work[s] to demonstrate life-affirming human connection amid chaotic violence" (Rubaii 2020, 213).

The study of trust in emergencies needs to recognize such trust without confidence or close connection and understands it as the emergent form of human relationship based on divergent interests, circumstantial affection and doomed togetherness. Especially in the face mask purchasing process, volunteers repeatedly expressed their distrust for the sellers in China. On the one hand, they strived to test the face mask samples using their professional knowledge and good connections. On the other hand, they chose to pay higher prices as a signal of trust for the sellers. To some extent, they were betting on the sellers' greed for the completion of a good cause. A new kind of relationship building is formed based on offering or being offered trust without much assurance, a possibility for "opening up new freedoms for others" (ibid., 214) by considering extending the boundaries of one's role to give hope for the bigger group.

However, the Chinese community in Gainesville is not a fleeting entity. After the liminal stage of trust (see Lim this volume), it is important to analyze how the face mask donation as a rite of passage can help the cultivation of a trustworthy community. Drawing on ritual studies by van Gennep (1960) and Turner (1967), participating groups after the liminal stage of the extraordinary events would obtain transformative power to reform their identity and relations. The Mandarin-speaking group have been intentionally creating a new group identity, which relies remarkably on their language skills, intellectual competence, professional credentials and cultural knowledge. They relied on the professional knowledge of the pandemic and healthcare system, financial resources to manage and account for the donation, social connections in both the Chinese and American societies and learned capacity to bridge the two cultural worlds has been accumulated with moral acceptance and value judgment of the merits and drawbacks of the sometimes-conflicting cultural traditions.

Debates around face mask wearing and donation reveal the complex dynamics of how an immigrant group can gain trust and recognition in the age of deadly pandemics and fierce political contests. The global debates on various preventative measures including face mask wearing and social distancing policies present an urgent yet unpredictable situation. Ordinary citizens, both in the US, China and other places, would bear great doubt of the information and instructions given by health professionals or governmental officials. The issue of ethnic identity has been extremely sensitive in the immigrant lives. We were intrigued to notice that all volunteers avoided discussing the issue as carefully as we tried in the interviews. Interestingly the volunteers tended to regard the different attitudes toward face masks and the indifferent response of some hospital staff as "cultural" and "educational" issues rather than ethnic or political chasms.

In this case, knowledge making, risk response and identity shaping depend much more on compassionate thoughts and moral judgments than ever. Trust is essential to what we argue is the compassionate knowledge making strategy in risk situations like COVID-19 pandemic. It refers to the fact that when people are confused easily by the heated debates even among renowned scientists, they would rather choose to rely on their own trusted information sources and respond with their own social responsibilities. They would make compassionate decisions of what to do for the best of their loved ones and close environment despite reserving different views on such practices.

In Gainesville, the face mask donation team were well aware of people's doubts on face mask wearing. Several volunteers interviewed admitted to us that early in the pandemic, even some medical professionals were not taking the face masks seriously. Instead of getting into a science, cultural or political "war" with other community members, the donation team focused on doing the common good for the whole community. On Facebook and Twitter, the face mask donation group repeatedly advocated for the use of face masks not only for personal health, but for the protection of the medical staff and of people's close contacts – the ones that people would be most concerned about during crises. The team relied on moral values of kinship ties, family wellbeing and social responsibility built on social trust to interpret and encourage the adoption of preventative measures. As one volunteer admitted to us, although some staff still did not care to wear face masks even at work, they expressed gratefulness for the donation and chose to wear one when possible. Science may not make one wear a face mask, but caring concerns often do.

It is in this sense that we further argue the community itself is also in a constant process of formation. Anthropological studies on community risk response and disaster recovery have long pointed out the contingency of community (Barrios 2014). They pay close attention to how the disaster-induced changes of political, economic and social circumstances and resources make communities rise and fall (Barrios 2014; Hoffman 2020; Oliver-Smith 1986). The Chinese community represented by Huagen is a historical product of the reformed political climate, economic collaboration and cross-cultural communication in China and the US since the late 20th century. The development of the Gainesville Chinese community witnesses the changing dynamics within the mainland Chinese immigrants as they grow from students to staff, professors to professionals. The generational, educational and economic characteristics have distinguished the Gainesville Mandarin-speaking group from other Chinese immigrant communities formed in previous times and in other places.

The make-up of the Gainesville community has also experienced radical changes as it is developing into a college town with large influx of Asian professionals. The careful community cultivation efforts have conclusively led to the success of the face mask donation.

Conclusion

The Gainesville Chinese community's emergency response to the COVID-19 pandemic showcases that a trusted and efficient community-based organization is an essential force to unite and utilize local resources in trying times. The chapter reveals that building trust during a crisis may always be enunciatory and dependent on the contingent and fleeting articulation of divergent interests, affection and togetherness. Enunciatory trust characterizes trust in liminality, and asks researchers to analyze the multiple and often cross-boundary intensions and happenstance that may lead to solidary and group action in emergent situations.

If the face mask donation is regarded as a rite of passage for the Huagen Chinese community in their endeavor of building social trust in their host community, the chapter further examines how the Chinese immigrant community can survive and thrive among the public health and social crises during and after the COVID-19 pandemic. The cultivation of a community's trust takes great patience, determination and careful planning. The chapter discusses how Huagen Chinese Language School gained their reputation and trustworthiness in the local community in the past 20 or so years. We argue that trust building requires both the development of confident and reliable relationships as well as the establishment of a community of socioeconomic resources and shared values.

The chapter explores the trust and distrust of the science of face masks, the Chinese as "virus carriers" and China-made PPE during the COVID-19 outbreak in the US. With the rising populist and right-wing nationalism inside the US since the outbreak of pandemic, Chinese immigrants have been impelled to further defend their legitimacy, values and national membership among the doubts and accusations of the face masks as well as the origin of the coronavirus (Zhang 2021). To cope with the COVID-19 pandemic, collective risk response depends more than ever on compassion and mutual care to promote common sense making and group action (Williams 1998). Trust is the cornerstone of such a compassionate relationship.

This chapter contributes to the understanding of risk response in the modern risk society where scientific reasoning and political agendas are greatly challenged by unforeseen and unmanageable threats. It argues that culturally embedded knowledge making and community practice of caring can help override gaps in times of crises when the authority of and trust for science, professionalism and the government are profoundly contested. Trust building in times of crisis essentially becomes a culturally informed practice. Therefore, healthcare practice and emergency response need to be (and have always been) interpreted and embodied in particular ethical values, interpersonal relations and historical consciousness in order to promote the mutual understanding of collective action.

Notes

1 Ziying You is the corresponding author.

2 The research is supported by China's National Social Science Fund Major Project (20&ZD152). Qiaoyun Zhang's part of research is also supported by UIC Research Grant with No. of R202048 at BNU-HKBU United International College, Zhuhai, PR China, Guangdong University Innovation and Enhancement Project with No. of R5202004 and The Joint Research Project of Guangdong Philosophy and Social Science Foundation with No. of R202116.

References

Barrios, Roberto. 2014. "'Here, I'm not at ease': Anthropological Perspectives on Community Resilience". *Disasters*: 329–350. doi: 10.1111/disa.12044.

Douglas, Mary. 1986. *Risk Acceptability According to the Social Sciences*. London: Russell Sage Foundation.

Douglas, Mary, and Aaron Wildavsky. 1983. *Risk and Culture: An Essay on the Selection of Technological and Environmental Dangers*. Berkeley: University of California Press.

Fortun, Kim. 2001. *Advocacy after Bhopal: Environmentalism, Disaster, New Global Orders*. Chicago: University of Chicago Press.

Hoffman, Susanna M. 2020. "'The Worst of Times, the Best of Times': Toward a Model of Cultural Response to Disaster". In *The Angry Earth: Disaster in Anthropological Perspective*, 2nd Edition, edited by Susanna M. Hoffman and Anthony Oliver-Smith, 141–156. London: Routledge. doi: 10.4324/9780203821190-17.

Holton, R. 1994. "Deciding to trust, coming to believe". *Australasian Journal of Philosophy* 72 (1): 63–76. doi: 10.1080/00048409412345881.

Jimenez, Alberto Corsın. 2011. "Trust in anthropology". *Anthropological Theory* 11(2): 177–196. doi: 10.1177/1463499611407392.

Levi, Margaret. 2015. "Trust, Sociology of". In *International Encyclopedia of the Social & Behavior Sciences*, 2nd edition, edited by James D. Wright, 664–667. Elsevier Ltd. doi: 10.1016/B978-0-08-097086-8.32162-6.

Levi, Margaret, and L. Stoker. 2000. "Political trust and trustworthiness". *Annual Review of Political Science* 3: 475–507. doi: 10.1146/annurev.polisci.3.1.475.

Mohl, Raymond A. 1995. "Asian Immigration to Florida". *The Florida Historical Quarterly* 73: 261–286. doi: 10.4324/9781351143127-14.

Oliver-Smith, Anthony. 1986. *The Martyred City: Death and Rebirth in the Andes*. Albuquerque: University of New Mexico Press.

Rayer, Stafan. 2017. Demographic Factors Driving the Growth of the Asian Population in Florida. Web article: https://www.bebr.ufl.edu/articles_publication/demographic-factors-driving-the-growth-of-the-asian-population-in-florida/

Rubaii, Kali. 2020. "Trust without Confidence: Moving Medicine with Dirty Hands". *Cultural Anthropology* 35 (2): 211–217. doi: 10.14506/ca35.2.03.

Turner V. 1967. *The Forest of Symbols: Aspects of Ndembu Ritual*. Itaca: Cornell University Press.

van Gennep, A., 1960. *The Rites of Passage*. University of Chicago Press, Chicago.

Williams, Melissa. 1998. *Voice, Trust, and Memory: Marginalized Groups and the Failings of Liberal Representation.* Princeton: Princeton University Press.

Zhang, M. (2021). Writing against "mask culture": Orientalism and COVID-19 responses in the West. *Anthropologica* 63(1): 1–14. https://doi.org/10.18357/anthropologica 6312021327.

10 Who to trust?

International migration risks and responses to the COVID-19 crisis in Mexico and Central America

Laurent Faret[1], *Olga Odgers-Ortiz, María Teresa Rodríguez López and Álvaro Caballeros*

Introduction

In this chapter, we reflect on the ways in which the COVID-19 pandemic disrupts the trust/distrust systems that prevailed in the migration corridor of Central America, Mexico and the United States. The general question that guides this chapter is: how is the trust/mistrust relationship structured and produced in a migratory context? Five specific questions are derived from this general question: how do migrants decide whom to trust? What are their decision-making criteria in risk situations, in migratory contexts characterized by a multiplicity of risks? How are the diverse representations of risk transformed in the context of the COVID-19 pandemic? How are criteria of trust/distrust being (re)defined?

Studies of transnational migration between Mexico and the United States have emphasized the role of networks in the mobility and settlement practices of migrants, which evolve from affective and material ties between the place of origin and the place of destination. The concept of transnational community precisely emphasizes the role of reciprocity networks for the circulation of resources of different kinds, so that migrants can maintain the relationship between their land of origin and the host country (Capone and Mary 2012: 31–33). On the other hand, the transnational social field paradigm has shown how migrants combine ways of being and belonging in specific contexts (Levitt 2001; Levitt and Glick Schiller 2004). These forms of belonging undoubtedly involve the permanence of strong social ties based on trust (Tilly 2007). In this field of study, ethnographic studies that have emphasized cooperation networks for the maintenance of ceremonial life and the support of families in the places of origin occupy an important place (D'Aubeterre 2005; Hirai 2009). The relationships of trust and the networks established at different scales are fundamental for the undertaking of migratory projects. In this chapter we are interested in showing that the crisis caused by the SARS-CoV-19 pandemic has had a disruptive effect on the postulates of the theory of migratory networks.

To answer these questions, we started analyzing empirical data collected over more than a decade through research on migration processes in the Central America/Mexico/US corridor (Odgers and Campos 2014; Alarcon

DOI: 10.4324/9781003291220-10

et al. 2016; Odgers 2020; Faret 2018, 2020; Rodríguez 2017, 2018; Caballeros 2018) as part of different projects financed by academic institutions in Mexico (COLEF, CIESAS), Guatemala (USAC) and France (University of Paris, IRD). Regarding the COVID period, we conducted on-site and online observation in shelters in the border city of Tijuana, Baja California, in Mexico City, in the southern states of Veracruz, Chiapas and the Mexico–Guatemala border region. Workshops with officials and migrants were also conducted in some places after the COVID-19 outbreak, especially in Tijuana and Mexico City. We additionally reviewed government policies and migration dynamics through media sources and reports. Although our analysis focuses on the Central America/Mexico/United States corridor, we believe these experiences can shed light on other migratory contexts.

We begin this chapter by discussing the trust/distrust dialectic in dialogue with previous literature. The second section describes how this dialectic is structured in migratory contexts along the corridor of Central America, Mexico and the US. In the third section we analyze how this dialectic has been disrupted by the outbreak of the COVID-19 pandemic. Finally, we discuss these results and suggest that new "danger figures" are created, drawing on the fear of contagion exacerbated by the pandemic.

The trust/distrust dialectic

Trust from a systemic perspective

Classical approaches are useful to understand how practical decisions are made by migrants on a daily basis: this helps us to understand how they decide who to trust. We believe that these approaches also help to understand the role of faith, a subjective factor that helps migrants to cope with adversity. From a systemic perspective, trust is considered a basic fact of social life (Luhmann 2005:5). For Luhmann, it is a mechanism for reducing social complexity, since it offers present assurances to future planning and orientations. From this perspective, for people in mobility, trusting some specific actors broadens the possibilities of action in the present, orienting toward a future that, although it remains uncertain, becomes trustworthy (Rodríguez 1996: XXIII). Trust can also concern the environment, not only people; it can also refer to the confidence in the effective functioning of the system (Rodríguez 1996: XXIV).

Faith designates the act of regarding something as worthy of credit; that is, that which is believed and which is expressed in a set of beliefs (Odero 1995: 165). Religious faith is a type of faith in the divinity, in the transcendent; it must be distinguished from a non-religious vital attitude that is also related to the act of believing: to put faith in something. Certain beliefs constitute vital bets, tinged with hope for a future project (168). Trust serves to reduce uncertainty about the behavior of other people (Odero 1995: 36) while accepting the risks involved, within limits and specific expectations (49). This is why trust can more easily turn into distrust than distrust into trust, since if a certain threshold is crossed, trust is lost (Rodríguez 1996: XXIII). In the Mexican migration context, it is common for people in mobility to turn to public institutions, migration authorities and other actors working with migrant populations. But loss of trust is frequent, as people face indifference, corruption, excessive bureaucracy and often the violation of their human rights (REDODEM 2019). Moreover, the analysis of the systemic relationship of trust and mistrust is not limited to this scale; it also involves individuals and the various formal and informal collectives that mobile people may encounter during their journeys, including the trust/mistrust relationship created among the migrants themselves. Finally, the transcendental level goes beyond the individual, network and institutional levels of trust and constitutes a general framework for the expression of hope. For Luhmann, trust is based on hope; since migrants do not have sufficient information to guarantee the success of a risky enterprise, they voluntarily overcome this information deficit by mobilizing a form of confidence in the fact that they can succeed. We suggest, then, that it is precisely in this void that faith in God or a transcendent being is placed, since trust is part of a system of values and pre-existing subjective dimensions.

The trust/distrust relationship as a dialectical process

Trust is defined in terms of positive assured expectations regarding the behavior of others, and distrust in terms of negative assured expectations regarding the behavior of others. By "assured positive expectations", Lewiki, et al. (1998: 439) refer to belief, the propensity to attribute virtuous intentions and the willingness to act based on another person's behavior. Conversely, by "assured negative expectations" they refer to fear; the propensity to attribute sinister intentions and the desire to protect oneself from the effects of another's behavior. Both trust and distrust imply movements toward certainty: trust, toward expectations of things viewed as positive; distrust, toward expectations of things to be feared (Lewiki, et al. 1998: 439).

Following Lewiki et al., we consider that trust and distrust are not static, since in every space-time context, there are factors pressing toward the growth or decline of trust, while other factors contribute to the growth or decline of distrust. In other words, trust and distrust are separate but concomitant; they vary throughout individual experiences, in various specific situations, in the different facets of complex interpersonal relationships (Lewiki, et al., 1998: 440). This variable and contingent dimension is characteristic of migratory trajectories; while strong levels of trust are generated in certain people and institutions, distrust in others is also generalized through lived experiences and through the information transmitted through different media and communication means. It is also possible for parties to trust and distrust each other to varying degrees. Interpersonal and social relationships are dynamic and often unpredictable.

We argue that migration contexts are fraught with mixed and multiple conditions that challenge people's ability to handle the complexities of simultaneous trust and mistrust. For this reason, we share the need to develop an understanding of the dynamics of relationships of trust and mistrust, which specifically anticipate conditions of ambivalence (Lewiki, et al. 1998.: 454).

Trust as social knowledge

Anthropology has shown that trust in institutions is one of the greatest strengths of society. Consequently, public distrust is indicative of social crisis, with the concomitant result of a breakdown of solidarity, cooperation and moral responsibility (Corsín 2011). Public and private institutions intervening in the management of migration in Mexico intend to transmit trust through ethical discourses that endorse contemporary values, such as respect for human rights, free mobility and the request for refuge (shelters, organizations of civil society, COMAR,[2] INM[3]). However, responsibility dissipates in the social whole, which translates into a dissipation and bifurcation of the subjects of social trust (Corsín 2011, citing Max Gluckmann 1972).

It is important to underline the significance of family networks when the subjects are outside their places of origin. During the migratory trajectory, migrants tend to trust family members and kinship relations much more, assuming that these are more trustworthy than strangers, consequently creating a well-defined network of social relations (Gurak and Caces 1992). These trusting relationships reduce uncertainty and vulnerability and tighten social ties to the extent that they enforce and return expectations of trustworthiness. Family has been interpreted as the key institution providing the basis of trust for collective action among immigrants entering the United States: family capital shapes independence and trust relationships in a world where the immigrants are strangers (Cook 2001: XIX). However, we consider that this dimension of trust provided by family and social networks is crossed by a permanent distrust of the "other". In places of transit and destination, the "other" is conceived as a latent threat; and this perception may be accentuated in the current pandemic context.

The stigmatization of the "other"

Wacquant (2009) points out that the criminalization of the urban poor – a category in which we can place migrants crossing Mexican cities – leads to the categorization of the public spaces they pass through as dangerous. This happens to Central American migrants in Mexico, partly because of their own irregular status. Additionally, in the context of the COVID-19 pandemic, they are also catalogued as potential carriers of the virus. In other words, there is a dissociation between those who have their place in the local community – including certain types of migrants who are considered trustworthy – and those who are considered risk carriers. Therefore, theories of "risk" must take into account the process by which suspicion arises, but also the reverse phenomenon, trust as the privilege of being above suspicion (Heyman 2009: 1).

According to Mary Douglas (1973), encounters that are considered dangerous carry with them a symbolic charge. The ideas of contamination are related to social life; that is, they express a general view of the social order. A contaminated person has developed some wrong condition or simply crossed a line that should not be crossed; this displacement triggers danger to others (Douglas 1973: 105). Migrants are stigmatized because of their otherness: they are poor, foreign, undocumented and potential disease carriers. In the context of the pandemic, stigmatization becomes more evident. Despite all this, people in mobility or entrapment move in the risk society (Beck 2020). For Beck, the dynamics of the risk society begin throughout the progressive processes of modernization and individualization, where human beings are forced to resolve their lives and their social ties. The concept of risk involves actions and decisions (Beck 2020: 175). Migrants make the decision to take a series of risks (deportation, violence, illness and even death) motivated by the desire to build a future different from their present.

Construction of attitudes toward risk, and trust/distrust patterns in migratory contexts

Migratory condition as an exacerbating factor in the trust/distrust dialectic

Whether made up of migrants from Central America or asylum seekers from Africa and other parts of the world, contemporary migratory flows through Mexico often include people who flee from structural violence, sometimes extreme (Odgers 2020; Faret 2020). Risk does not begin with migratory displacement: risk is present at its source and is part of the individual experience. It is associated with poverty, violence, climate change and the consequences of failed political systems that do not focus on the causes of emigration (Collyer 2010; Morales 2008). In this context, migrants are led to face risks both in their places of origin and along migration routes, as elements of what has been described as a *continuum of violence* (Faret 2020: 45). This deplorable situation is accentuated by the progressive reinforcement of mobility control (reinforcement of border control, borders externalization, more restrictive protocols for requesting asylum) and an increasingly dangerous immigration system, disrupted by organized crime (Leutert 2018; Faret et al. 2021).

In migratory routes, risk is not an abstract fear. It is tangible: the risk of running out of money on the journey, of not having anywhere to sleep or anything to eat, the risk of being extorted, kidnapped, raped, beaten or murdered (REDODEM 2019). Despite this, fieldwork evidence shows that in the most adverse conditions, migrants maintain confidence that they will be able to reach their destinations, that everything will be okay in the end. This confidence, which is rooted in faith and nurtures trust building, is probably one of the most salient characteristics of migrants' attitudes. This faith-nurtured trust is closer to positioning than a rational calculation. In this sense, it is of a more abstract nature – in opposition to tangible risks – and remains associated with an interpretation of the world sustained in religious orientations. Without recognizing this, it would be impossible to understand the perseverance of individuals and the reproduction of migratory flows.

Thus, in a path where surviving is constantly at stake, our first observation is the exacerbation of the dialectic between abstract trust and concrete distrust, toward actors and institutions with which migrants interact along the way. As detailed in the following section, this dialectical relationship is expressed in different ways, in various places and times.

The trust/distrust dialectic at four levels of analysis

To analyze the trust/distrust dialectic in this migratory field, we distinguish four levels of analysis: the individual, constituted social groups and networks, the institutions and the transcendental level (related to faith).

At the individual level, there are three main dimensions to take into consideration: information, identity and experience. The amount (and nature) of information that one has about the other can be direct – for example, relatives traveling together – or indirect – as when acquaintances put migrants in contact with persons they may find on their journeys. But getting in contact with others activates other resources to decide whom to trust: to establish trust/distrust relationships with strangers, the possibility of identifying with the other is crucial. Trust will be more easily developed with a person with whom a sense of ethnic, national, religious or gender identity is shared. In other words, the perception of identity and "otherness" becomes paramount. However, strangers can become new figures of trust through experience. As proposed by Lewiki, it is possible to identify how trust/distrust relations vary along individual experiences, in diverse specific situations and in different facets of complex interpersonal relationships (Lewiki et al. 1998: 440). During the journey, many experiences – both positive and negative – are shared with strangers. Shared experiences create bonds of affection and trust; however, these links are sometimes ephemeral insofar as they are circumstantial and the trajectories and routes are widely diversified. Finally, at this level, it is important to mention the importance of confidence in one's own ability to respond to unforeseen events that arise on the journey as well as to adapt to the conditions of the destination. Trust in one's own capabilities becomes another kind of trust that is relevant at the individual level. Self-confidence is an important factor when making the decision to migrate; it is part of the subjectivation processes involved in the migration experience. The process of building confidence is mediated by personal history and by meanings associated with gender, social class, culture and socialization processes (Sevillano and Escobar 2011: 225). However, self-confidence is not an acquisition that remains stable, since it is dynamic and changing according to circumstances and life experiences.

At the level of constituted social groups (NGOs, shelters, legal advice organizations) and networks, migrants' reactions are ambivalent, due to their heterogeneity. The reactions and relationships of migrants with respect to established social groups (NGOs, reception centers, legal advice organizations and networks) are very diverse and largely ad hoc. Migrants trust social groups and networks because they need to. In order to continue moving, they need this support, so the question is not to trust or not to trust, but how to choose the most reliable social group or network. Or, following Luhmann, decisions are taken as a mechanism for reducing social complexity by offering present assurances to future planning and orientations (Luhmann 2005: 5). There would be no migration without trust at this level, but it remains, however, a cautious trust. Trust serves to reduce the element of uncertainty about the behavior of other people (Luhmann 2005: 36), but accepting the risks involved within limits and in proportion to rational and specific expectations (Luhmann 2005: 49). Migrants go to shelters when they have nowhere to sleep, but it is not until positive interpersonal relationships have been established with other sheltered migrants or with shelter staff that they start truly trusting this space. Likewise, migrants seek the free services of volunteer doctors, but do not fully trust their diagnoses and prescriptions: they often reinterpret, adapt or abandon them (Olivas, Odgers, Bojorquez, forthcoming).

At the institutional level, distrust prevails. There is fear of the legal action of the institutions, which could detain and deport them in compliance with current legislation. But there is also the fear of inefficiency and corruption of immigration agencies, security agents or even public health providers, which could put them at risk of being unjustly detained or extorted. This is similar to Corsín's scenario, where public distrust is indicative of a social crisis (Corsín 2011). However, the concomitant result of a breakdown of solidarity, cooperation and moral responsibility anticipated by Corsín is relative, since distrust in institutions coexists with trust in other domains, as indicated in relation to the levels of the individual and social groups/networks. Even more, with the fourth level or dimension of trust analyzed here, it is related to the confidence in a transcendent being that will not let them down.

Confidence in God is undoubtedly a significant trait of the trust/distrust system in this migratory context. In this case, this is an expression of confidence supported by value systems: faith and religion. Faith is understood not only as believing in God – or a transcendent entity – but also as believing in the contractual bond between God and the faithful (Prescendi 2010); hence the confidence that God will not abandon those who believe in him. That it, faith, is produced on an abstract/transcendental level, but has practical consequences boosting confidence in a positive outcome of migratory journeys, thus creating a "positive-but-cautious" predisposition toward others. This structural and subjective dimension of trust that corresponds to the realm of the spiritual, pre-existing migratory systems, turns out to be a key element to understand why, despite all the adversities, migrants keep confidence in being successful. It is important to repeat that while it is true that faith is sustained in the transcendental realm, it has crucial implications for worldly decision-making.

In sum, while the trust/distrust system is heterogeneous and ever-changing in the individual and social groups/networks spheres, in the institutional sphere distrust prevails. Following Lim (*in this special issue*) we identify in the Central America/Mexico/US corridor a differentiated trust system, where a low system trust coexists with a high particularized trust, producing higher social group trust relative to system trust; trust enactment can be identified through multiple local responses competing with political and medical responses and with multiple risk sources and blame targets. In this sense, Lim's model is useful to understand the functioning of this system. Nevertheless, we consider it necessary to incorporate the fourth sphere presented above – faith or transcendent trust – to understand why migrants continue moving along this long and dangerous route.

Trust production: experience, prestige and contracts

Throughout the migratory journey, people will require a set of goods (food, clothing, medicine) and services (accommodation, information, means of communication and transportation) essential to survival and to continuing the journey. It is then necessary to trust in order to survive and keep on going along the route. Thus, the crucial question is: who to trust? In choosing whom to trust – where to sleep, which coyote to cross the border with, which medical service provider to approach, etc. – people in migrations are guided by three main trust production mechanisms.

First, there are the relationships that have been built through direct interaction, either with migrants from their village or region of origin whom they meet along the way, or with strangers with whom they have had the opportunity to interact. Some contacts have been previously established through migratory networks giving migrants confidence that they will arrive at a certain place where there is someone trustworthy who will support them by providing accommodation or temporary employment. Second, they trust actors who hold forms of prestige, which are built and transmitted through migratory networks. This aspect is central, for example, when choosing a guide or *pollero*, or when purchasing identity documents: they would prefer a service provider that has a reputation for being honest, empathic and efficient. Third, migrants would prefer services that are guaranteed by some form of contract – verbal, in most cases – that allows knowing more precisely what to expect.

Finally, it is important to remember that the decision on whom to trust is not permanent, either because a trusted individual or group betrays the trust placed in them, or because they are no longer present in this migratory corridor. This was the case of community guides or *polleros*: with the process of strengthening border control, the prices of undocumented crossing increased, making this activity more attractive to criminal groups. As a consequence, local or regional mafias displaced community *polleros*. Although up to now we have focused on mobile individuals as subjects, it should also be noted that historically migrants have been constructed – by the states, the media – as figures of danger. By stigmatizing the migrant, not only are additional obstacles imposed along the way, but above all, the establishment of interpersonal relationships along the routes through which they travel is made difficult. This aspect will be discussed further.

Migration and the trust/distrust nexus in pandemic times

In the context of the COVID health crisis, transformations in social interactions between migrants and different actors in the countries of presence (transit or settlement) are important issues. As shown above, people on the move engage on a daily basis in relations with diverse types of actors, in formal or informal ways, for short or long periods and according to different grades of trust/distrust representation. If the COVID-19 situation has had an impact on all of these interactions in a broad sense and for everyone, these transformations are particularly important for migrants, who have as their main objective to continue their geographic mobility at a time when the suppression of mobility is being advocated as a strategy to contain the advance of the pandemic (Bojorquez et al. 2021; Coubes et al. 2020; US CBP 2021). In various Latin American countries, confinement paralyzed the ongoing processes of regularization of the migrant population and the processing of asylum claims. Borders were also closed and, in some cases, even militarized. Proof of this was the militarization of the border between Peru and Ecuador to prevent the passage of migrants as a way of preventing the spread of the contagion. These measures have contributed to leaving large numbers of irregular migrants defenseless and in need of international protection (Herrera 2021: 106–116). Something similar happened at the Mexico–Guatemala border and on the border between Guatemala and Honduras. But at the same time, the multiplicity of risks that migrants face locates the pandemic as "just another risk" among many others and not necessarily as the one of highest concern. However, the pandemic also transforms the perception of other people about migrants as risk carriers, disrupting the trust/distrust dynamic.

The importance of the COVID-19 pandemic in the region must first be highlighted. Beginning in the first months of 2020, the pandemic situation caused a health crisis in Mexico and Central America, with lockdown restrictions starting in March. This was quickly accompanied by a socioeconomic crisis, as all activities were affected and ordinary life was challenged by the risks of infection as well as by the limitations on travel and economic operations (Gonzalez et al. 2021). The Latin American economy contracted by 7.7% and almost three million companies closed in 2020 due to the pandemic. In addition, the region accounted for nearly 28% of deaths from COVID-19 worldwide, despite the fact that only 8.4% of the world's population lives in the region, according to the UN economic commission for the region in a report in which it urges maintaining emergency aid at least during this year to alleviate the social impact of the crisis (CEPAL 2021).

If no strict measures of confinement were applied in the region, the general instructions from the authorities of Mexico, Honduras, El Salvador and Guatemala have been to stay at home and to limit activities to what was essential to domestic supply and could not be postponed. In one year, the COVID-19 pandemic was responsible for more than 208,800 deaths in the four countries of Mexico, Guatemala, Honduras and El Salvador.[4] Mexico alone had 2.2 million confirmed COVID-19 cases and 196,000 deaths, with a significant level of saturation of hospital facilities. Moreover, the migration routes from south to north across Mexican territory go through different local environments with high degrees of pandemic impact, such as, for example, the Mexico City region or in the Pacific Coast states from Nayarit to the Mexico–US border in Tijuana, which happened to be an additional factor of worry for people on the move. The restrictions due to the pandemic situation, the closures of facilities and the worsening of economic conditions formed a set of barriers and worries for people on the move, creating additional difficulties on top of those previously existing; socioeconomic vulnerability of migrants has increased throughout 2020 and early 2021 (Wilson and Choy 2020; Bojorquez et al. 2020).

The conditions of risk in migratory contexts have been reshaped with modes of intervention by public authorities that have become even more restrictive, with the closure of borders at the national level and containment orders at the local level. The way civil society organizations intervene has also become more complex, as they have been under the pressure of health measures and also of migrants' deteriorating situations. As local observations show, the forms of trust that persist in these risk contexts are the most private ones – when available – such as family networks of local or transnational scope, trust in NGOS that are locally constituted and hold everyday interactions during the pandemic period, or other small groups formed on a temporary basis, as in the case of shelters that have kept receiving new migrants.

We consider two perspectives to explore the trust/distrust dynamic in pandemic times. From a phenomenological perspective we observe how COVID-19 has been integrated, in migrants' experiences, into the panorama of risks disrupting the trust/distrust nexus. In this way, we consider that international migrants have run into the pandemic in their trajectories according to places and specific temporalities. From a subject's perspective, we highlight how migrants' representation has been subject to a reconfiguration by other social actors, modifying the trust/distrust granted to them as subjects in mobility. In this sense, we pay attention to how society in a pandemic situation "has encountered migrants" once again, and how the construction of figures of danger has been (re)built in pandemic – and probably post-pandemic – times.

Acting migrants, new configuration and relative perceptions of risk

Trust/distrust relationships were transformed in the context of the pandemic in terms of risk perceptions, and social interactions were affected. In the context mentioned in the preceding section, COVID has come to be inserted as one risk among many others, not necessarily as a danger over and above the other challenges. This is not to say that, for a moving population, the restrictions of the pandemic context and its widespread immobilization have not had important effects; they actually have. But in migrants' own expressions, the COVID situation was one more matter of concern, in addition to those that existed before, and that people have to deal with in the course of their mobility. With the pandemic, migrants encounter the same actors, but their roles are changing in terms of what they may offer or what has to be feared from them.

As other studies have shown, the vulnerability of migrants has increased with complications related to the concrete expressions of immobilization and disrupted journeys in the context of the pandemic. Among the main features, the most significant one – and the one that has been most widely publicized – is border closures, although those closures have had different expressions in the region. The

Mexico–US border remained closed for 20 months, beginning in March 2020 (Gonzalez et al. 2021), while border-crossing activities in the Central American isthmus were suspended for shortened periods. It should be noted that the border between Guatemala and Mexico was closed on March 18, 2021, for a one-month period, with a governmental decision taken with direct reference to prevention of the spread of COVID (EFE 2020). It should be highlighted that the announcement came on the same day that the US government announced it would share 2.5 million doses of vaccine with Mexico, leading observers to interpret the border closure as yet another element of the externalization of borders under pressure from the US and long-standing geopolitical influences in the region (Faret 2018).

The shutdown of institutions, activities and migration procedures has also been deeply resented and badly experienced, especially in the case of applicants for international protection status. As for the population as a whole, the saturation of hospitals and health care centers has been a matter of concern. The shutdown of transportation services and related infrastructures (buses and transfer stations, airplane flights and airports) has had an impact on mobility, in parallel with labor market contraction and job losses in the places of temporary residence or along the migration routes, leading to precarious economic situations. On another matter, the closure and control of communities to prevent the entry of strangers and migrants was part of local strategies in some places in Guatemala or Mexico, alongside the creation of centers for returnees where people had to go through a quarantine period before they could go back home. As an extreme form, troubles and protests occurred in some temporary centers of attention for returnees and their nearby surroundings (for example in Guatemala, Veracruz and Chiapas). In some communities, aversion and stigmatization of returnees in Mexico and the three Central American countries were noted, leading to rejection by part of the local population upon the arrival of returnees. Additionally, in Guatemala and elsewhere, there have been cases where local indigenous authorities have closed their communities, forbidding access to all returning migrants or other people coming from abroad, for fear of them infecting the local population (Álvaro Caballeros, personal observation).

Interactions with CSOs and shelters

Civil society organizations have remained a central element during the pandemic. As the historical "trusted actor", these organizations remained active in pandemic times, but with significant new modalities or restrictive rules. Restrictions on the activities of civil society organizations are of impact: some shelters remained closed for several months, all of them applied specific rules when opened, and others did not let people get out as they used to do. The specific security measures have sometimes meant that shelters continued to receive asylum seekers or refugees in an installation process, but remained inaccessible for some periods to people in transit looking for a few days' rest in their journey from south to north, as they were seen as potentially contagious. This was the case, for example, in the shelters located in the cities of Acayucan and Coatzacoalcos, Veracruz. Other shelters, such as the one located in Guadalupe La Patrona, municipality of

Amatlán de los Reyes, Veracruz, set up a space separate from the main facilities in order to provide lodging for migrants in transit, but the dining room remained closed. In the course of the pandemic, rapid changes were noted: initially, restrictive measures were established (for example, no way for the people who are hosted to leave the shelter at any time), but gradually the rules grew less stringent or were no longer observed, specifically when the urge to get out and find some economic activities appeared as a matter of primary importance for residents. As an example, at the beginning of the pandemic and the lockdown, a significant number of migrants preferred to leave the shelters in Tijuana or Mexico City to look for another place to stay. But progressively, in the face of the need to work and to send remittances, people began to leave the shelters, and migrants assumed the idea of coming out of shelters and taking risks (Bojorquez et al. 2021). Entry/exit restriction protocols were seen as a burden in many cases, as control over movement and action was lived as an additional and unnecessary constraint in regard to direct needs (and in some way with regards to age, as migrants often see themselves as less exposed than older people) (Bojorquez et al. 2021).

Inside the shelters, dialectics of trust/distrust were not absent either, as collective spaces had to be shared. As observed in the fieldwork, migrants sometimes stated that they were not so afraid when they went out on the street, but feared contaminating others when they came back in. Moreover, a certain amount of trust is implicit in staying in a shelter and using the communal spaces of daily life. Periods of pandemic have challenged this trust, generating at times moments of tension and conflict within the shelters. In some cases, distrust toward the shelters is also mentioned, as their restrictive rules have been seen as an additional element of suspicion, and migrants have felt that they were "in the eye of the authorities", as they had to give a lot of personal information with the worry that this would be transmitted to the local or national authorities. In the case of doctors and nurses visiting and helping people in shelters with medical issues, the ones that were previously seen as bringing useful service and support are now transformed into those who come to limit, to prevent and to scare.

Interactions with institutions

In pandemic times, the mistrust of state institutions previously mentioned remains high, and concerns all institutions at levels from local to national, and at borders as well as at reception structures in diverse urban areas or along the routes. To some extent, the shutdown of activities and the restrictions in reception and regularization procedures have been interpreted as a new obstacle and as discriminatory, reinforcing the feeling of mistrust. As an example, the "integration centers for migrants" – launched in 2019 at the northern border of Mexico (in Ciudad Juárez, Tijuana and Mexicali) – did not appear to be relevant options for migrants, as they were seen as new detention centers. The spatial isolation from the local population and from possible economic opportunities was interpreted as "set apart" strategies. The mistrust is not only toward the state but also toward the major international organizations, like IOM, which was among the organizations in charge of these centers. Another expression of clear mistrust has been the way recent caravans of migrants have been received: since the beginning of the pandemic, previously tense relations with national authorities at borders have worsened. In January 2021, the Guatemalan government answered to the Central American "caravan" of migrants with military action to impede entry into its territory, arguing that the "situation puts the population at risk in terms of health", as the Guatemalan official in charge of migration issues said to the media.[5] At the same time, Mexico also reinforced the military presence at its southern border. Many civil organizations reported excessive use of force to physically detain individuals, which was interpreted as a rejection of migrants at a time when the reasons to migrate remain high.

Interpersonal interactions (with other migrants, local population and communities of origin)

Since the COVID crisis cannot be considered a homogeneous period, it is difficult to characterize social interactions as a whole during this period, just as it is difficult to consider the evolution of migrants' situations in the Central and North American region as uniform, due to quite different socioeconomic conditions. Nevertheless, a common factor in terms of interactions with others would be that people in mobile situations had to go out in search of resources: they could hardly stay at home as recommended by the authorities, even assuming that this idea of a home was applicable to people on the move. Like other sectors of the population with little economic income, they had to continue to engage in outdoor activities and contact with others during the pandemic. The particularity here is that interpersonal relationships took place for migrants in less familiar environments than for sedentary populations, so that the type of relationship of trust or distrust played a more important role. As mentioned earlier, the data collected during the fieldwork led to the conclusion that the pandemic did not represent a greater fear than insecurity, violence or unemployment. Carvel considers himself fortunate to have had an employer who asked him to continue working during confinement:

> I was lucky to have an understanding employer. During the peak of the pandemic he paid me even though I wasn't working. Then he asked me to start working again and I said yes. I was lucky to have a job!

But conditions have changed due to unfamiliar situations, with a decrease in direct interactions between actors and new forms of mistrust that migrants must face. Two examples of this can be stressed. The first one is a mistrust that was not present prior to the crisis, the one expressed in the communities of origin in the face of the return of migrants. Observations and indirect information converge on the cases of local communities that "closed" themselves to the return of migrants (whether the return was voluntary or resulted from expulsion), for fear of importing the virus. Adverse reactions were recorded, as fear and uncertainty in the face of possible contagion rendered the people arriving from abroad as a matter of concern, regardless of whether they were close relatives or not. Faith, a Cameroonian refugee working at an OSCs shelter, explains: "There are many people to help now, because of COVID! Many black people were fired from their jobs or asked to leave the flat they lived in, because they are seen as COVID carriers". Such interactions raise a new and important dimension of mistrust: the migrant who had for years been the one supporting the community (through remittances, investments in the place of origin, networks that allow others to follow his path), suddenly becomes a threat. The feeling that the community has "turned its back" on people who have had to seek economic opportunities outside their place of origin is strong in these cases, as is a sense of betrayal.[6]

Another example concerns the issue of trust in terms of the quality and reliability of the information that circulates among people on the move, and how some information networks have changed. As is well known, a great deal of information circulates and is central to migration plans, such as which routes and border crossings are safer, how to access documents or how to find economic resources. With fewer direct contacts during the pandemic, many people had to rely on information provided by lesser-known people. This is the case with the many networks supported by communication technologies and mobile devices (WhatsApp or Facebook groups, for example, or institutional pages), but with no guarantee as to the identity of the person generating the information, its reliability or the validity of what is learned. At the same time, direct information from relatives with recent experiences was scarce or irrelevant due to the ongoing changes and immobility of many, reducing the help these traditional and trusted contacts could provide. In analytical terms, physical and social interaction with relatives, known as the usual basis of trust systems, is being challenged by the growth of fewer interpersonal networks with a high capacity to adapt to changing situations but with less certainty about the veracity of information sent from a distance. Although not new, this process may have been more far-reaching during the pandemic period.

Constructing "danger figures" in times of pandemics: new issues

There are two aspects in which the impact of the pandemic appears really significant as part of a changing panorama: the construction of the migrant as a figure of danger, due to the possibility of being a vector of contagion, and the incorporation of COVID-19 into the geopolitical scenario of the region. We consider that these two analytical lines should be further explored in greater depth, based on the following reflections that could offer possible avenues for future research.

The body of the migrant: representations, fears and attitudes

In the construction of the trust/distrust dialectic among and toward the migrant population, the body has always played a preponderant role, both as a factor of vulnerability and as a threat. Thus, understanding corporeality is a key point for understanding trust/distrust relationships, whether the integrity of the migrant's own body is at stake in the face of violence or health risks (Vearey et al. 2020) or whether it is reified in exploitative labor relations (Della Puppa 2019; Holmes 2013). In the social construction of fear of the migrant, the migrant's body has occupied a critical place, whether in relation to sex, ethnicity, sexual orientation and youth identities, among others (Parrini et al. 2007; Valenzuela et al. 2007). As an example, the discursive plasticity with which young Central American migrants are often described is meaningful, as they may be referred to as workers or asylum seekers, or criminals because – in some cases – their bodies are tattooed (Navarro 2007: 191–193). Central American youth have been surrounded by a "delinquent aura" (Monsiváis 2007: 333); e.g., Honduran women are negatively perceived and associated with sex work (Rivera 2019). In the representation of the migrant as a "figure of danger", mobility is alluded to as a threat, and he/she is presented as one who "invades" the space of "others" with his/her material presence.

Our field observations lead us to argue that the COVID-19 pandemic is deepening this process of stigmatization and marginalization: while health authorities mandate confinement and immobility as a strategy to contain the spread of the virus, migration tends to be perceived as a risk and a transgression of the official discourse. This is far from the perception of other forms of mobility, such as trade or tourism, that are seen as social practices that have to be supported during the crisis time and for which the fastest possible recovery is sought. During the pandemic, existing prejudices about migrants as "bodies on the move" increased, just when the immobilization of bodies was presented as a global health strategy. By being on the move, the migrant becomes the transgressor *par excellence*, the emblematic figure of risk: the pre-existing cultural dimensions of mistrust persist, but a supplementary layer is added: since the risk is anchored to the biological entity that circulates, the body that moves becomes a new threat as a possible disease carrier.

It is true that this dimension had already been present. For example, in relation to HIV transmission, the body of the returned migrant was constructed as a figure of danger, as had happened previously with homosexuals (Deane et al. 2010). But unlike HIV, the importance of restricting mobility for the control of the COVID-19 pandemic has the consequence of spreading fear even to those who "pass through". In this sense, there is a convergence in the current construction of the migrant as a figure of danger, with what happened in other historical periods (Piret and Boivin 2020).

The construction of the migrant as a figure of danger, as a possible carrier of the virus, can be observed both in the places through which migrants pass and in the institutions in charge of mobility management (e.g., COMAR restricts in-person attention and transfers some procedures to the virtual environment; court appointments for migrants in MPP are suspended). In the case of communities of origin, the relevance of the physical dimension is even more evident. For example, in certain indigenous populations in Guatemala, inhabitants decided to prohibit access to returning migrants from the United States or Mexico for fear of contagion (Álvaro Caballeros, personal observation in Huehuetenango). However, telephone communications and contacts through social networks have intensified, and remittances continue to flow without obstacles to these same communities, underlying that the problem is the body. This flow of communications and exchanges allows the maintenance of feelings associated with the experience of trust; these feelings are fundamental to creating and maintaining interpersonal relationships that provide a certain emotional and affective tranquility (Sevillano and Escobar 2011: 228). In the course of 2022 – particularly with the advance of vaccination campaigns – a progressive loss of the centrality of COVID in the risk landscape is likely to be observed, it is also likely that the stigmatization of the migrant body will persist in places of transit and destination.

COVID, migration and (geo)politics

In terms of what may outlast the health crisis, another important avenue for future research is the geopolitical dimension of the migratory processes and the way the main actors interact in the region. How these actors proceed could lay the foundation for new relationships of trust and distrust in mobility matters, a crucial point in the current context. As is known, the issues at the crossroads between a health crisis and geopolitical relations are numerous in the region, and observers of the COVID-19 period have paid attention to different elements, such as the diffusion of the pandemic, the movement restrictions it produces and the geopolitical tensions over vaccination matters. Many of those challenges arose in a context of controlling mobile populations and pre-existing concerns about transit migration from third countries. On the trust/distrust dialectic, some elements are of specific interest, as they highlight the evolution of relations between nation-states and international migrants at different scales. In this sense, the COVID period may be seen as a continuation of previous processes as well as a catalyst of new trends, with conditions and forms of action whose scope is difficult to measure at present but could be longer in extent than the pandemic period itself.

In a similar way to the perspective about the body, the construction of a "figure of danger" in times of crisis appears to be a useful analytical perspective. In the region, the rhetoric of crisis is nothing new; it has been an element of public policies of contention, externalization of border controls and restrictive measures for migrants, for the past decade at least (Zaiotti 2016; Villafuerte 2011). In many ways, the process of immobilization that characterizes the COVID period is reminiscent of what has happened in other moments, such as the "crisis" of minors stranded at the Mexico–US border in July 2014, or the caravans in Central America and through Mexico in 2018 and 2019. In these moments, national authorities produced a discourse based on distrust of mobile populations, questioning the legitimacy of their movement and their refugee claims; this became the basis for new plans to tackle undocumented migration. The Mexican "Programa Frontera Sur" in 2014 was part of this strategy for Mexico (Isacson et al. 2017; Ribando 2019), and the US Migrant Protection Protocols (MPP) – better known as the "Remain in Mexico" program – were launched in reaction to the migrant caravans in 2019 (Paris and Díaz 2020). Those measures increased operations at borders and along routes, leading to a significant rise in apprehensions by migration authorities in the region (Faret et al. 2021).

In pandemic times, the risk of COVID contagion and mobility restrictions becoming intertwined as geopolitical issues affecting the ongoing control of mobile populations is rather high. Actually, the pressure during the last months from receiving countries to generate immobilization policies at national borders and in transit countries is very comparable to earlier episodes. The military response to new caravans in Guatemala in January 2021 and the closure of the Mexican southern border in March 2021 are examples of this trend. They come at a time when negotiations on vaccine supply are a leading issue, and they render the migration issue an element of bilateral negotiation, as has so often been the case in the past in the region (Caballeros 2018; Faret 2018). Also – and although the new Biden administration in the US has shown more positive signs than the previous one on the migration issue – the southern border of the United States is again subject to restrictive measures for migrants, associated with the risk of contagion. In 2020, the Trump administration clearly used COVID-19 as a justification to turn away or immediately expel asylum seekers. This policy, activated under public health code Title 42, remains in effect today, with exceptions for unaccompanied children, some families and those impacted by the PPT.

Another indication of the production of figures of danger and distrust toward mobile populations in pandemic times is the criminalization of activities related to traditional migration systems and their actors. As reported in this chapter, migration systems have historically been built on strong relations of trust between individuals, families and local actors in the migration process, including transporters, local coyotes (smugglers) and diverse intermediaries. Many of them are today under the fire of criminalizing discourse; traditional migratory networks that provide support and resources to migrants have been criminalized and fought and the traditional coyote is now presented as a trafficker. If some of those actors have been associated with organized crime and human trafficking, there is a certain ambiguity that tends not to distinguish between the types of activities undertaken or the purpose of the migration entrepreneurs. As an example, the US embassy's media campaign launched in Guatemala and El Salvador in 2021 – aimed very directly at dissuading people from going north – particularly emphasizes the role of intermediaries, seen as criminals spreading false information and putting people at risk. In any case, first estimations of the impact of the COVID crisis on trafficking activities report that the immobilization process primarily benefits criminal actors in the medium and long term, as the militarization of borders, the reduction of safe and legal routes and measures of control are likely to increase the vulnerability of migrants at any point in their journey (Bird 2020). Once again, there is a growing body of evidence that warns of a pandemic situation being instrumentalized to produce new forms of vulnerability, global distrust and increase of risk. But at the same time, the effects of the pandemic and the social and economic crisis in Central America will continue putting people on the move.

Conclusion

Trust emerges as a mutual co-involvement of interests between parties, i.e., agreements between potentially trustworthy individuals who have reciprocal expectations distributed in a variety of tangible and intangible ways. That is why it belongs both to the realm of intersubjectivity and to that of inter-objectivity. In its anthropological dimension, trust emerges as an epiphenomenon of social knowledge, so it can be considered as a "cognitive category" (Corsín 2011), a way of knowing the world. This is important because it refers to the understanding of the meaning that subjects give to their actions; it alludes to the interpretation of personal and collective experiences, which is of specific interest in a changing context resulting from a crisis situation.

As argued throughout this chapter, the trust/distrust dialectic is an important dimension of the functioning of migration systems, and crisis situations challenge it. Three main areas are important when analyzing the processes of trust/distrust construction in the migratory experience. First, trust is to be considered as part of a value system, and as such, as a subjective dimension that pre-exists and encompasses social interactions. In the case of migrants moving through the Central America/Mexico/United States migration corridor, religion and, more comprehensively, faith, are central, in the sense that they transcendentally enable the migratory enterprise. Second, trust in a migratory situation is produced in parallel by the contribution of social and interpersonal networks as well as confidence in a person's ability to adapt to unexpected events and circumstances. In the latter case, trust is fragile and contingent, and therefore more uncertain in the context of a crisis. Third, distrust of institutions is widespread, and tends to increase with the barriers to movement and restriction of mobility associated with the health crisis. This distrust is less pronounced, however, with respect to religious and civil society institutions that run shelters for migrants along the migration corridor. Moreover, the construction and maintenance of trust is a multifactorial process, and, in many ways, migrants must make decisions under conditions of vulnerability – sometimes extreme – in order to move forward. Being exacerbated with the arrival of the COVID-19 pandemic, the situation of marginalization or liminality has come together with increasing risks, obstacles to mobility and stigmatization processes toward migrants.

However, while mitigation measures have in some ways exacerbated the adverse conditions faced by migrants, what is observed is more a worsening of a pre-existing situation than a profound transformation of the trust/mistrust production system. For migrants, COVID-19 is just one more risk they face on their journey. And it is not necessarily the one risk that instills the greatest fear in them. The impact is important, however, because during pandemic times, as social inequalities have increased, so have the "resources" of the population in vulnerability been reduced. Trust is one of the resources that has been diminished.

Notes

1 Laurent Faret is the corresponding author.
2 COMAR (Comisión Mexicana de Ayuda a Refugiados) is the governmental institution in Mexico responsible for processing applications for refugee status.
3 INM (Instituto Nacional de Migración) is a unit of the government of Mexico dependent on the Secretariat of the Interior that controls and supervises migration in the country.

4 Data on March 18, 2021, from Johns Hopkins Bloomberg School of Public Health.
5 *El Pais*, January 17, 2021, "Guatemala frena por la fuerza la caravana de migrantes que se dirige hacia México", https://elpais.com/mexico/2021-01-17/guatemala-frena-por-la-fuerza-a-la-caravana-de-migrantes-que-se-dirige-hacia-mexico.html.
6 To have a comparative context would take us back to the 1980s and 1990s, with the fear of the spread of HIV in the regions of origin.

References

Alarcón, Rafael, Luis Escala & Olga Odgers Ortiz. 2016. *Making Los Angeles Home. The Integration of Mexican Migrants to the United States*, University of California Press.

Beck, Ulrich. 2020. "La teoría de la sociedad del riesgo reformulada", Polis, México, UAM, 16(2): 171–196. Available at: https://polismexico.izt.uam.mx/index.php/rp/issue/view/45/showToc

Bird, Lucia. 2020. *Smuggling in the Time of Covid-19. The Impact of the Pandemic on Human-smuggling Dynamics and Migrant-protection Risks*. Report of the Global Initiative Against Transnational Organized Crime, https://globalinitiative.net/wp-content/uploads/2020/04/GIATOC-Policy-Brief-003-Smuggling-COVID-28Apr0930-proof-4.pdf

Bojórquez, I., Odgers-Ortiz, O. & Olivas-Hernández, O. L. 2021. "Psychosocial and mental health during the COVID-19 lockdown: A rapid qualitative study in migrant shelters at the Mexico-United States border", *Salud Mental* 44(4): 167–175. https://doi.org/10.17711/SM.0185-3325.2021.022

Bojorquez, Ietza, Infante, César & Vieitez, Isabel. 2020. "Migrants in transit and asylum seecers in Mexico: an epidemiological analysis of the COVID-19 pandemic", MedRxiv preprint. May 13, 2020. https://www.medrxiv.org/content/10.1101/2020.05.08.20095604v1

Caballeros Herrera, Álvaro. 2018. "Análisis regional de las dinámicas de movilidad, dispositivos de seguridad y políticas migratorias", *Estudios Interétnicos* 29: 123–138.

Capone, Stefania & Mary, André. 2012. "Las translógicas de una globalización religiosa a la inversa", in: *En sentido contrario. Transnacionalización de religiones africanas y latinoamericanas*. (Kali Argyriadis, Stefania Capone, Renée de la Torre & André Mary, coords.) México: CIESAS, 27–46.

Collyer Michael. 2010. "Stranded Migrants and the Fragmented Journey", *Journal of Immigrant and Refugee Studies*, 23 (3): 273–293.

Comisión Económica para América Latina y el Caribe (CEPAL). 2020. *Panorama Social de América Latina*, 2020 (LC/PUB.2021/2-P/Rev.1), Santiago, 2021.

Cook, Karen S. 2001. "Trust in society", in: *Trust in Society* (Cook, Karen S., ed.), New York: The Russell Sage Foundation Series on Trust, Vol. II, xi–xxvii.

Corsín Jiménez, Alberto. 2011. "Trust in anthropology", in *Anthropological Theory* 11(2): 177–196. https://journals.sagepub.com/doi/10.1177/1463499611407392#

Coubès, M. L., Velasco, L. & Contreras, O. 2020. *Poblaciones vulnerables ante COVID-19*. El Colegio de la Frontera Norte. https://www.colef.mx/estudiosdeelcolef/migrantes-en-albergues-en-las-ciudades-fronterizas-del-norte-de-mexico/

D'Aubeterre, M.E. 2005. "San Miguel Argángel, un santo andariego: Trabajo ceremonial en una comunidad de transmigrantes del estado de Puebla", in *Relaciones*, XXIV (103): 18–50.

Deane, K., Parkhurst, J. & Johnston, D. 2010. "Linking migration, mobility, and HIV", *Tropical Medicine and International Health* 15(12): 1458–1463. DOI: 10.1111/j.1365-3156.2010.02647.x

Della Puppa, F. 2019. "Bodies at Work, Work on Bodies: Migrant Bodies, Wage Labour, and Family Reunification in Italy", *Journal of International Migration & Integration* 20, 963–981. https://doi.org/10.1007/s12134-018-00644-x

Douglas, Mary. 1973. *Pureza y peligro. Un análisis de los conceptos de contaminación y tabú*. Madrid: Ed. Siglo XXI.

EFE. 2020. "Guatemala cierra fronteras tras confirmar seis contagios y una muerte por COVID-19", *Agencia EFE*, mars 16th, Available at: https://www.efe.com/efe/america/sociedad/guatemala-cierra-fronteras-tras-confirmar-seis-contagios-y-una-muerte-por-covid-19/20000013-4197293

Faret, Laurent. 2018. "Enjeux migratoires et nouvelle géopolitique à l'interface Amérique latine - Etats-Unis", *Hérodote* 4(171): 89–105.

Faret, Laurent. 2020. "Migrations de la violence, violence en migration. Les vulnérabilités des populations centraméricaines en mobilité vers le Nord". *Revue Européenne des Migrations Internationales* 36 (1): 31–52.

Faret, Laurent, Anguiano María Eugenia & Rodríguez Luz Helena. 2021. "Migration Management and Changes in Mobility Patterns in the North and Central American Region", *Journal on Migration and Human Security* 9 (2): 63–79.

Gluckman, Max. 1972. "Moral crises: Magical and secular solutions. The Marett lectures, 1964 and 1965", *The Allocation of Responsibility*: 1–50.

Gonzalez, E., Harrison, C., Hopkins, K., Horowitz, L., Nagovitch, P., Sonneland, H & Zissis, C. 2021. *The Coronavirus in Latin America*. AS/COA (American Society / Council of the Americas), February, 2021. https://www.as-coa.org/articles/coronavirus-latin-america

Gurak, Douglas T. & Fee Caces. 1992. "Migration networks and the shaping of migration systems", In: *International migration systems: A global approach* (Kritz, M., L. Lim and H. Zlotnik eds.). Oxford: Oxford University Press, Clarendon Press, 150–176.

Herrera, Gioconda. 2021. "Migraciones en pandemia: nuevas y viejas formas de desigualdad", *Nueva Sociedad* 293: 106–116

Heyman, Josiah McC. 2009. "Risque et confiance dans le contrôle des frontières américaines", *Politix, Revue des sciences sociales du politique* 87: 21–46.

Hirai, S. 2009. *Economía política de la nostalgia: Un estudio sobre la transformación del paisaje urbano en la migración transnacional entre México y Estados Unidos*. México, Casa Juan Pablos, 405 pp.

Holmes, Seth. 2013. *Fresh Fruit, Broken Bodies: Migrant Farmworkers in the United States*, Univ of California Press, 234 pp.

Isacson, Adam, Hannah Smith & Meyer, Maureen. 2017. *La frontera sur de México. Seguridad, migración centroamericana y políticas estadounidenses. Informe de investigación*. Mexico: WOLA. https://www.wola.org/es/analisis/informe-de-wola-la-frontera-sur-de-mexico-seguridad-migracion-centroamericana-y-politicas-estadounidenses/

Leutert, Stephanie. 2018. "Organized Crime and Central American Migration in Mexico", *Report from the LBJ School of Public Affairs*. Austin, The University of Texas, 40 p.

Levitt, P. 2001. *The Transnational Villagers*. University of California Press, 395 pp.

Levitt, P. & Schiller, N. G. (2004). "Conceptualizing Simultaneity: A Transnational Social Field, Perspective on Society", *The International Migration Review* 38(3): 1002–1039.

Lewicki, Roy J., Mcallister, Daniel J. & Bies, Robert J. 1998. "Trust and distrust: New relationships and realities", *Academy of Management Review* 23(3): 438–458.

Luhmann, Niklas. 2005. *Confianza*. UIA-Anthropos: Epaña.

Monsiváis, Carlos. 2007. "Los enigmas de la Mara Salvatrucha (carta abierta en forma de epílogo)", in: *Las maras. Identidades juveniles al límite.* (Valenzuela et al. eds.) México: UAM-COLEF-JP, 323–333.

Morales Gamboa Abelardo. 2008. "Migraciones, regionalismo y ciudadanía en Centroamérica", in: *Migraciones en el sur de México y Centroamérica* (Villafuerte & García, eds.), Mexico: Porrúa/Unicach/Cámara de Diputados, 49–75.

Navarro, Javier. 2007. "La construcción de un enemigo: seguridad, maras y derechos humanos de los jóvenes", in: Las maras. Identidades juveniles al límite. (Valenzuela et al. eds.) México: UAM-COLEF-JP, 187–208.

Odero, J. M. 1995. "Sobre la categoría de 'fe religiosa'", *Revista de ciencias de las religiones*: 163–172.

Odgers Ortiz, O. 2020. "The perception of violence in narratives of central migrants at the border between Mexico and the United States", *Revue Européenne de Migrations Internationales* 36: 1. DOI: 10.4000/remi.14452

Odgers Ortiz, O. & Campos Delgado, A. 2014. "Suspended in the mouvement: Waiting periods and spaces for Mexicans Deported from the US", *Revue Européenne de Migrations Internationales* 30: 2. DOI: 10.4000/remi.6922

Paris Pombo, María Dolores & Díaz Carnero, Emiliano I. 2020. "La externalización del asilo a la frontera Norte de México: protocolos de protección al migrante", in *Migraciones en México: fronteras, omisiones y transgresiones. Informe 2019* (Red de Documentación de las Organizaciones Defensoras de Migrantes eds.) México: REDODEM. https://redodem.org/wp-content/uploads/2020/09/REDODEM_Informe_2019.pdf

Parrini, R., Castañeda, X. & Magis, C. et al. 2007. "Migrant bodies: Corporality, sexuality, and power among Mexican migrant men", *Sexuality Research and Social Policy* 4: 62. https://doi.org/10.1525/srsp.2007.4.3.62

Piret, J. & Bovin, G. 2020. "Pandemics throughout history", *Frontiers in Microbiology* 11. https://www.frontiersin.org/articles/10.3389/fmicb.2020.631736, https://doi.org/10.3389/fmicb.2020.631736.

Prescendi, F. 2010. "Foi", in *Dictionnaire des faits religieux* (T. Azira & Hervieu-Léger). PUF, 388–391.

REDODEM (Red de Documentación de las Organizaciones Defensoras de Migrantes). 2019. "Procesos migratorios en México. Nuevos rostros, mismas dinámicas", *Informe 2018*, México: Servicio Jesuita a Migrantes, 247 p. [online]. http://redodem.org/wp-content/uploads/2019/09/REDODEM-Informe-2018.pdf

Ribando Seelke, C. 2019. *Mexico's Immigration Control Efforts*. Washington, DC: Congressional Research Service, https://fas.org/sgp/crs/row/IF10215.pdf

Rivera, Carolina. 2019. "Poder sobre el precario trabajo sexual femenino en la franja transfronteriza Chiapas-Guatemala", in: *Entre dos fuegos. Naturalización e invisibilidad de la violencia de género contra migrantes en territorio mexicano* (Hiroko Asakura & Marta W. Torres Falcón, coords.), México: CIESAS, 187–213.

Rodríguez, Darío. 1996. "Introducción", in: Confianza (Niklas Luhmann). México-Santiago de Chile: Universidad Iberoamericana-Ed. Antrhopos, VII–XVII.

Rodríguez, María Teresa. 2017. "Hondureños en la capital veracruzana. Anhelos y estrategias de migrantes en tránsito", *Migración: nuevos actores, procesos y retos* (Magdalena Barros & Agustín Escobar, coords.). México: CIESAS, 166–189.

Rodríguez, María Teresa. 2018. "Estar de paso. Trayectorias centroamericanas en el centro de Veracruz", in: *El territorio como recurso: movilidad y apropiación del espacio en*

México y Centroamérica (Odile Hoffmann & Abelardo Morales, coords.), San José: Costa Rica, FLACSO-IRD-LMI-Meso-UNA, 133–160.

Sevillano, Merlyn Johanna & Escobar, María Cénide. 2011. "Confianza-desconfianza en las relaciones conyugales de parejas transnacionales", *Prospectiva: Revista de Trabajo Social e Intervención Social* 16: 225–256.

Tilly, C. 2007. "Trust Networks in Transnational Migration", *Sociological Forum*, 22(1): 4–24.

U.S. Customs and Border Protection. 2021. *Nationwide Enforcement Encounters: Title 8 Enforcement Actions and Title 42 Expulsions 2022*. U.S. Customs and Border Protection. https://www.cbp.gov/newsroom/stats/cbp-enforcement-statistics/title-8-and-title-42-statistics

Valenzuela, José Manuel, Nateras Alfredo & Reguillo, Rosana (coords.). 2007. *Las maras. Identidades juveniles al límite.* México: UAM-COLEF-JP.

Vearey, J., Hui, C. & Wickramage, K. 2020. "Migration and Health: current issues, governance and knowledge gaps", in *World Migration Report*. DOI: 10.18356/9ea52c60-en

Villafuerte Solís, Daniel. 2011. "Políticas de seguridad y migración internacional en la frontera sur de México", in *Migración, seguridad, violencia y derechos humanos, lecturas desde el sur*, edited by Daniel Villafuerte Solís & María del Carmen García Aguilar. México: Miguel Ángel Porrúa-Unicach, 167–207.

Wacquant, Loïc. 2009. *Castigar a los pobres. El gobierno neoliberal de la inseguridad social*. Barcelona: Ed. Gedisa.

Wilson, Jania & Choy Gómez, Jorge. 2020. ¿Migrar con sana distancia? *Nexos*, 16/XI/2020: https://migracion.nexos.com.mx/author/jorge-choy-gomez/

Zaiotti, Ruben. 2016. *Externalizing migration management. Europe, North America and the spread of 'remote control' practices*. New York: Routledge.

Index

For Product Safety Concerns and Information please contact our EU representative GPSR@taylorandfrancis.com Taylor & Francis Verlag GmbH, Kaufingerstraße 24, 80331 München, Germany